The Celiabetic Kitchen

by
Gloria Moore

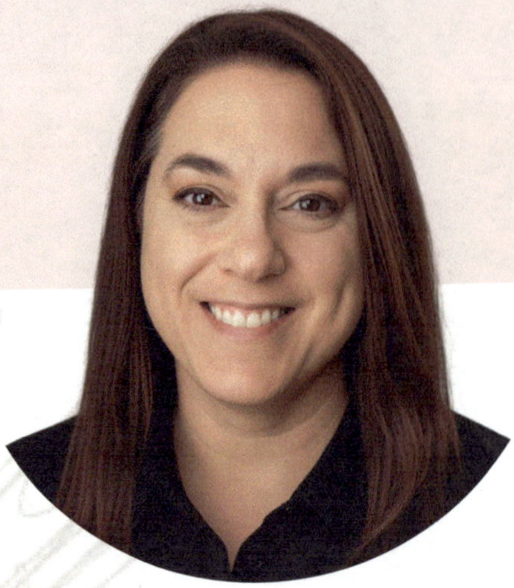

Greetings From the Author

Welcome, friends! My name is Gloria, and like you, I'm navigating the choppy waters of living with both celiac disease and diabetes. When people ask how I manage what they see as double dietary restrictions, I smile and tell them I've discovered something unexpected: these challenges have actually made me a better cook, a more adventurous eater, and surprisingly, someone who enjoys food more than ever before.

For me, when I couldn't rely on convenience foods or default to the same old recipes everyone else uses, I was forced to get creative. Then, when I understood how different ingredients affect my body, I started building meals with intention rather than habit. And when I finally mastered that perfect gluten-free, blood sugar-friendly version of my Mother's Coconut Cream Pie? Well, that victory tastes sweeter than any sugar rush ever could.

I'm not a nutritionist or a professional chef – I'm simply someone who loves good food and refuses to let dietary restrictions diminish that joy. Through years of kitchen experiments (some successful, others... educational), I've learned that the intersection of gluten-free and diabetes-friendly cooking isn't a barren wasteland of deprivation. It's actually a place where fresh ingredients shine, where spices and herbs take center stage, and where you discover that what your body needs and what your taste buds crave can absolutely be the same thing.

Whether you're managing celiac disease, diabetes, or both – or perhaps you're simply looking to reduce gluten and stabilize your blood sugar for other health reasons – this cookbook is your companion on the journey. Together, we'll prove that eating well with dietary restrictions isn't about what you're missing; it's about all the delicious possibilities you're about to discover.

Gloria Moore

The Celiabetic Mission

This cookbook is a true passion project, a self-published labor of love brought to life by an incredible circle of support. It began in my own kitchen and grew from there, nurtured by the generous encouragement of friends, the honest feedback of family, and the creative talents of colleagues and contributors. Every recipe, photo, and story within these pages is a testament to what a community can create together, and I am endlessly grateful for the village that helped make this book a reality.

That spirit of community is at the heart of everything this project stands for. Just as others supported me on my journey, I believe in paying that support forward. That is why this book is also a mission-driven effort to bring safe, nourishing food to those who need it most. We are proud to dedicate 10% of all proceeds to stocking food pantries across the United States with celiac-safe and low-glycemic products, partnering with amazing organizations to make a tangible difference.

By purchasing this book and reading its pages, you are stepping into that circle of support. Your purchase not only values the work of a self-published author but directly contributes to our Celiabetic mission. Thank you for being a part of this story and for helping us share the gift of safe, delicious food with others. To learn more and join the mission, please visit www.TheCeliabeticKitchen.com.

With over 3 million Americans managing celiac disease and 38 million living with diabetes—and significant overlap between these populations—The Celiabetic Kitchen addresses the fastest-growing intersection in special-diet cooking.

Medical and Nutritional Disclaimer:
This book is intended for informational and educational purposes only. The author is not a medical professional, registered dietitian, nutritionist, or certified diabetes educator. The recipes and dietary suggestions in this book are based on the author's personal experience with celiac disease and diabetes management and general wellness principles. They should not be used as a substitute for professional medical or nutritional advice, diagnosis, or treatment.

Important Health Warnings:

- Always consult a qualified healthcare provider, registered dietitian, or certified diabetes educator before making significant changes to your diet or lifestyle, especially if you have celiac disease, diabetes, pre-existing health conditions, dietary restrictions, or food allergies.
- Individual nutritional needs vary significantly based on age, weight, activity level, medications, and other health factors. The recipes in this book may not be appropriate for all individuals.
- Cross-contamination risk: Readers with celiac disease must verify all ingredients are certified gluten-free and take appropriate precautions to prevent cross-contamination in their kitchens.
- Blood sugar monitoring: Readers with diabetes should monitor their blood glucose levels closely when trying new recipes, as individual responses to foods can vary significantly.
- Nutritional information provided is approximate and based on specific brands and measurements. Actual values may vary depending on ingredients used.

While every effort has been made to ensure the accuracy of the information, recipes, and measurements in this book, the author and publisher assume no responsibility for errors, omissions, adverse reactions, or adverse effects resulting from the use of the recipes, information, or recommendations provided. Individual results may vary.

Ingredient Accuracy: Readers are responsible for verifying that all ingredients used are safe for their specific dietary needs and restrictions. Food manufacturers may change product formulations without notice. Always read ingredient labels carefully.

Liability Limitation: To the fullest extent permitted by law, the author and publisher disclaim all liability for any direct, indirect, incidental, consequential, or special damages arising from or in any way connected with access to or use of this book, even if advised of the possibility of such damages.

First Edition: 2025
Published By: Producers Publishing

Table of Contents

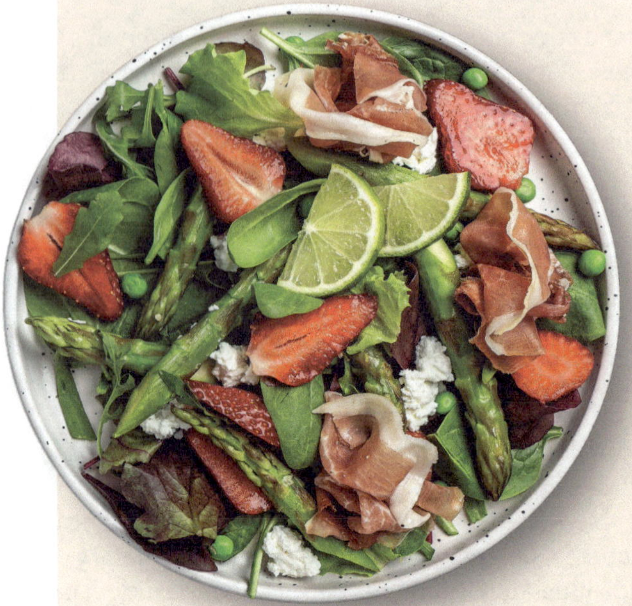

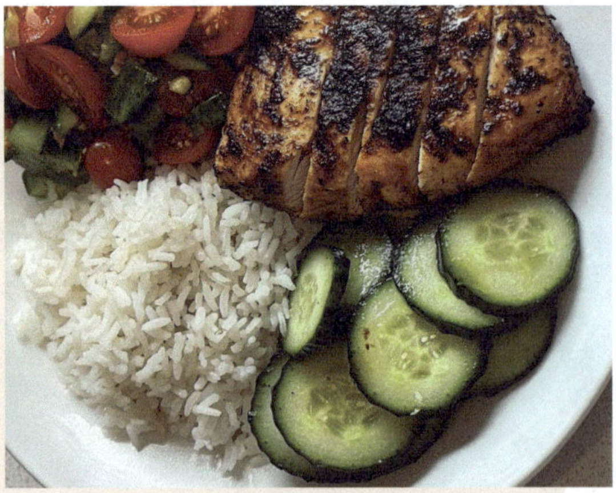

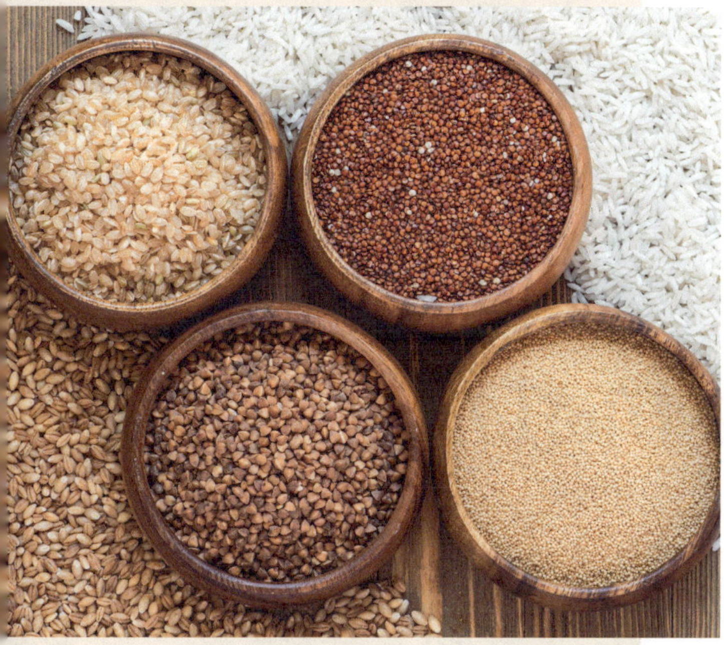

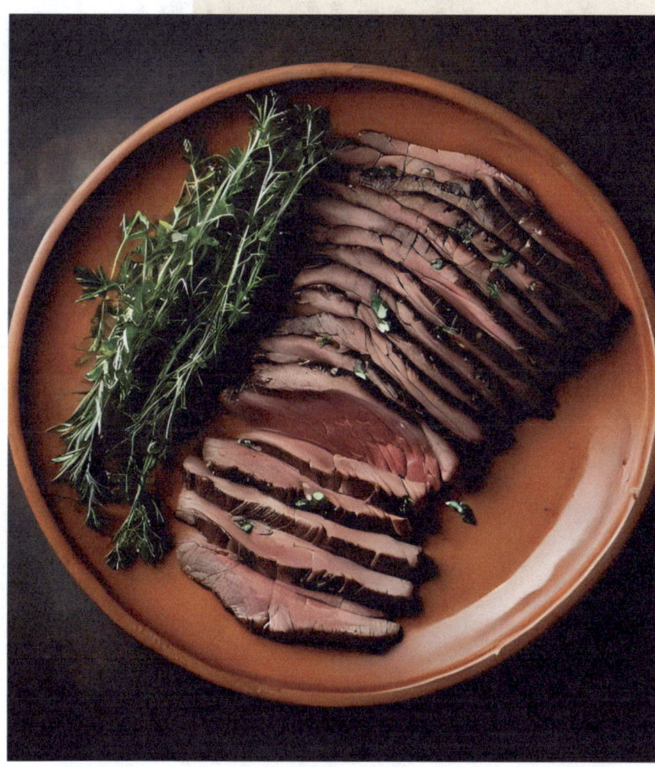

The Kitchen Confidence Motto:

"True freedom lies not in the absence of restrictions, but in the mastery of living well within them."

"Your diagnoses don't define you or limit your possibilities—they're simply new parameters within which creativity and joy can still flourish."

CHAPTER 01

Kitchen Essentials & Pantry Staples

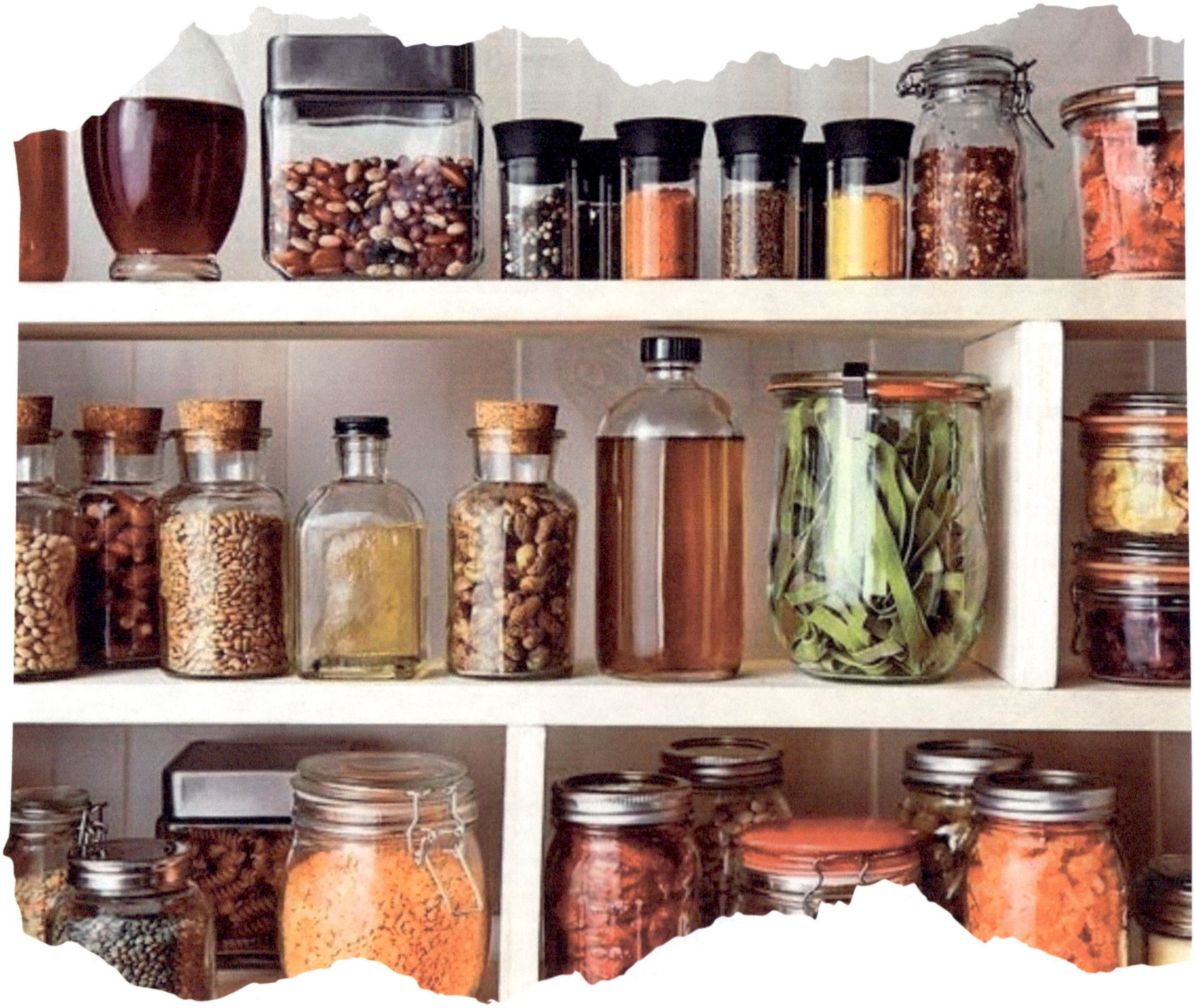

Building a well-stocked kitchen that serves both gluten-free and diabetes-friendly cooking doesn't require a complete overhaul of your pantry or a second mortgage. The key is understanding which staples will work hardest for you, offering versatility, nutrition, and blood sugar stability. This chapter focuses specifically on the foundational ingredients that appear often throughout this cookbook – the building blocks that make gluten-free cooking possible and diabetes management easier.

I've chosen to highlight three essential categories: gluten-free flours and baking basics that replace wheat-based ingredients, low-glycemic sweeteners that satisfy your sweet tooth without spiking blood sugar, and healthy fats that enhance both flavor and nutritional value. These aren't the only ingredients you'll encounter in this cookbook – far from it. As you explore the chapters ahead, you'll discover dozens of fresh vegetables, lean proteins, herbs, spices, and specialty ingredients that bring variety and excitement to your meals. But master these foundational staples first, and you'll have the confidence to tackle any recipe that follows.

This chapter will give you an overview of these essential ingredients with practical tips for shopping smart, storing properly, and understanding how each one contributes to both your health goals and your cooking success.

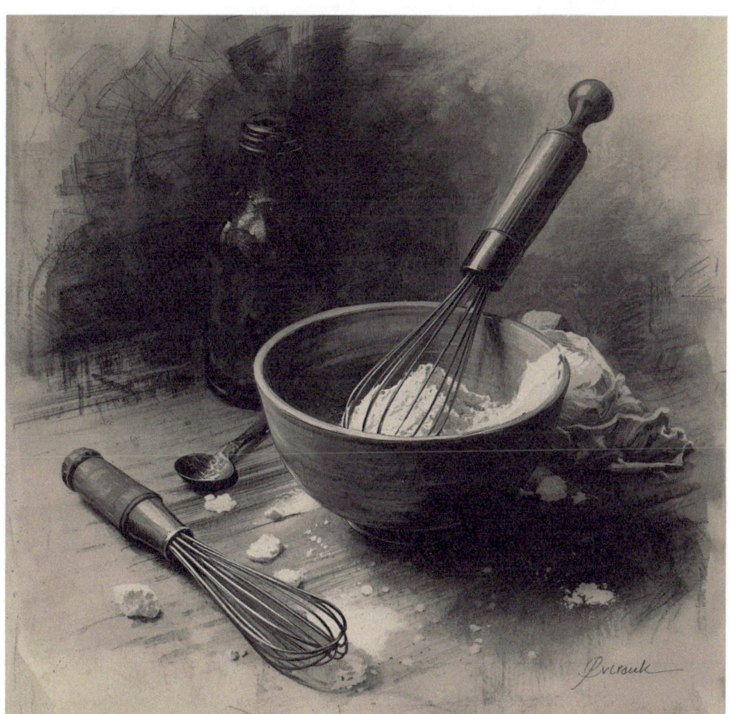

Gluten Free Flours

Almond Flour

Made from finely ground blanched almonds, almond flour is naturally gluten-free and rich in protein, fiber, and healthy fats. It provides a tender crumb and a slightly nutty flavor, making it ideal for cakes, cookies, and quick breads. Because it lacks gluten's elasticity, almond flour works best when combined with starches or binding agents like eggs or xanthan gum. Keep refrigerated or frozen to keep it fresh longer.

Coconut Flour

Derived from dried, ground coconut meat, coconut flour is highly absorbent and requires significantly more liquid than traditional flours. It adds a light coconut flavor and is rich in fiber, which can help moderate blood sugar spikes. Recipes typically use only a small amount, balanced with extra eggs or other liquids. Best stored in an airtight container in the refrigerator.

Brown Rice Flour

A mild, versatile staple in many gluten-free flour blends, brown rice flour provides a neutral flavor and a lighter texture. It's often used in combination with starchier flours to create balance in baked goods. Because of its whole grain content, it offers more fiber and nutrients than white rice flour. It does have a higher carb content and will need to be used sparingly to prevent blood sugar spikes. Store in a cool, dry place and use within six months for freshness.

Tapioca Starch (Tapioca Flour)

This starch is extracted from the cassava root and contributes chewiness, elasticity, and lightness to baked goods. While it doesn't add much nutritional value, it's a key player in replicating the structure and texture of wheat-based recipes. Overuse can cause gumminess, so it's typically blended with other flours.

Oat Flour (Certified Gluten-Free)

Ground from oats processed in gluten-free facilities, oat flour has a mild, slightly sweet flavor and contributes softness and moisture to baked goods. It's rich in soluble fiber, which supports blood sugar stability and satiety. Works well in muffins, pancakes, and cookies when blended with higher-protein flours.

Chickpea Flour (Garbanzo Bean Flour)

High in protein and fiber, chickpea flour adds structure, density, and a slightly earthy flavor. It works particularly well in savory recipes like flatbreads, fritters, and thickening sauces. Its nutritional profile makes it an excellent choice for balancing carbohydrates in gluten-free baking.

Low-Glycemic Sweeteners

Stevia (Pure Leaf or Liquid)

This incredibly potent natural sweetener is derived from the leaves of the Stevia rebaudiana plant. It offers a zero-calorie option with no impact on blood sugar levels, making it ideal for individuals managing diabetes or those seeking to reduce calorie intake. Stevia is about 200 to 300 times sweeter than table sugar, so it's important to start with tiny amounts and adjust gradually to achieve your desired sweetness. Be cautious of blends that contain added sugars or bulking agents, as these can negate its benefits.

Monk Fruit Sweetener

Sourced from the monk fruit, this sweetener provides a zero-glycemic solution with a cleaner, more neutral taste compared to stevia, which some people find has a bitter aftertaste. Although it tends to be more expensive, it's highly valued in desserts where the flavor of the sweetener is crucial. Its unique sweetness comes from mogrosides, compounds found in monk fruit, which offer sweetness without affecting blood sugar.

Erythritol

As a sugar alcohol, erythritol offers sweetness with minimal impact on blood sugar levels, making it suitable for diabetics or those on low-carb diets. It measures cup-for-cup like sugar, which simplifies substitution in baking recipes. However, while it generally works well in most recipes, consuming it in large quantities can cause digestive upset for some people, due to its incomplete absorption in the digestive tract.

Allulose

This is a rare sugar naturally found in small quantities in foods like figs and raisins. Allulose tastes and behaves remarkably similar to regular sugar, offering a satisfying sweetness with minimal impact on blood glucose levels. It measures cup-for-cup like sugar and browns beautifully, making it an excellent choice for baking. Although more expensive than other sweeteners, it is highly prized for its ability to produce the most authentic results in desserts and baked goods.

Unsweetened Applesauce

A natural sweetener that not only adds sweetness but also moisture to baked goods, making it a versatile ingredient for healthier baking. Choosing organic applesauce when possible ensures that you avoid pesticides and other chemicals, and always checking labels for added sugars is crucial. Its affordability makes it a budget-friendly option for those looking to reduce sugar intake while maintaining flavor and texture in their baked creations.

Pure Vanilla Extract

This aromatic extract enhances the perception of sweetness in recipes without adding sugar itself. Opting for pure vanilla extract over imitation varieties ensures a richer, more complex flavor, which can elevate the taste of baked goods and other sweet treats. Moreover, it offers subtle benefits for managing blood sugar levels, making it a valuable addition to any pantry.

Healthy Fats & Oils

Extra Virgin Olive Oil

This oil is renowned for its delicate flavor and versatility, making it ideal for low-heat cooking methods such as sautéing and light frying. It is also a popular choice for salad dressings, where its fruity and peppery notes can shine through, and for finishing dishes, adding a rich depth of flavor. To preserve its quality, purchase it in dark bottles that protect it from light, and store it in a cool, dark place away from heat. When selecting extra virgin olive oil, look for labels indicating cold-pressed and first-pressed for the best quality.

Avocado Oil

Known for its exceptionally high smoke point, avocado oil is an excellent choice for high-heat cooking techniques like roasting, frying, and sautéing. Its mild, neutral flavor means it won't overpower other ingredients, allowing the natural flavors of your dishes to come through. It's also rich in healthy monounsaturated fats and vitamin E, making it a nutritious option for everyday cooking. Keep it in a cool, dark place to maintain its stability and flavor.

Coconut Oil

This versatile oil is solid at room temperature, which makes it particularly useful in baking, where it can be used as a substitute for butter or shortening to achieve a flaky texture. Unrefined coconut oil imparts a distinct coconut flavor, ideal for tropical or sweet recipes, while refined coconut oil offers a neutral taste, suitable for savory dishes. Coconut oil is also highly stable, with a long shelf life, and can be used for medium-heat cooking.

Ghee (Clarified Butter)

Ghee is a staple in many traditional cuisines, prized for its rich, nutty flavor and high smoke point, which makes it suitable for frying and sautéing. It's lactose-free, making it a great option for those with lactose intolerance. Although ghee is more expensive than regular butter, it has a longer shelf life and does not require refrigeration, which can add convenience to your cooking routine. Ghee can also enhance the taste of Indian and Middle Eastern dishes, where its unique flavor profile is especially appreciated.

Sesame Oil

Commonly used in Asian cuisine, sesame oil adds a distinctive, nutty flavor to dishes. It's perfect for stir-frying and seasoning vegetables and meats. There are two types: light sesame oil, which has a mild flavor and is suitable for frying, and toasted sesame oil, which has a more intense flavor and is best used as a finishing oil or in dressings.

Peanut Oil

With its high smoke point, peanut oil is ideal for frying and deep-frying, providing a subtle nutty flavor that complements a wide variety of dishes. It is often used in Asian and Southern cooking and is particularly favored for frying foods like chicken and fish. Peanut oil is also high in monounsaturated fats, making it a healthier choice for heart-friendly cooking.

Smart Shopping Strategies

Transitioning to a gluten-free, diabetes-friendly kitchen doesn't mean you need to empty your shelves and start over. Instead, think of it as a gradual layering process—adding versatile, high-impact ingredients one at a time until your pantry naturally supports the way you want to cook and eat. This approach keeps things manageable for your budget and ensures you learn how to use each ingredient before moving on to the next.

A good first step is stocking the most flexible, everyday essentials. Brown rice flour, for example, is a dependable backbone for many gluten-free flour blends, while olive oil provides both heart-healthy fat and flavor for cooking and finishing dishes. Add in basic spices and seasonings you already enjoy—garlic powder, paprika, cinnamon, dried herbs—and you'll have the foundation to make ordinary meals both gluten-free and flavorful without stress.

Once you're comfortable with the basics, begin layering in specialty items like almond flour, coconut flour, and alternative sweeteners. These may seem expensive at first glance, but buying them in bulk online or at warehouse stores often lowers the cost significantly. Because these ingredients are nutrient-dense, you'll typically use smaller amounts in recipes than you would traditional wheat flour or sugar, which means they stretch further than expected. Storing flours like almond or coconut in the refrigerator or freezer also extends their freshness, ensuring nothing goes to waste.

It's equally important to remember that your pantry is meant to support—not replace—fresh cooking. Whole foods like vegetables, fruits, lean proteins, and legumes are naturally gluten-free and blood sugar-friendly, and they provide the bulk of your meals. Pantry staples simply make these fresh foods more versatile and satisfying. For example, a hearty vegetable soup becomes more filling when thickened with a spoonful of chickpea flour, and a basic grilled chicken dinner transforms into something special with a simple almond flour crust or a drizzle of good olive oil.

The final key is quality. Investing in the best versions of your staples pays off in flavor, nutrition, and efficiency. Pure vanilla extract may cost more than imitation, but you'll use less of it to achieve better results. Extra-virgin olive oil might feel like a splurge, yet it enhances everything from salad dressings to roasted vegetables. Over time, you'll find that choosing quality ingredients actually makes your kitchen more economical, because you'll waste less and cook more meals at home rather than relying on costly convenience foods.

By taking a step-by-step approach, you'll build a pantry that truly works for you—a collection of ingredients that makes weeknight dinners faster, special-occasion baking possible, and healthy eating feel natural rather than restrictive. When the shelves are stocked with the right essentials, you'll be prepared to create satisfying, nourishing meals without last-minute shopping trips or the stress of realizing you're missing a key ingredient.

CHAPTER 02

Understanding Your Ingredients

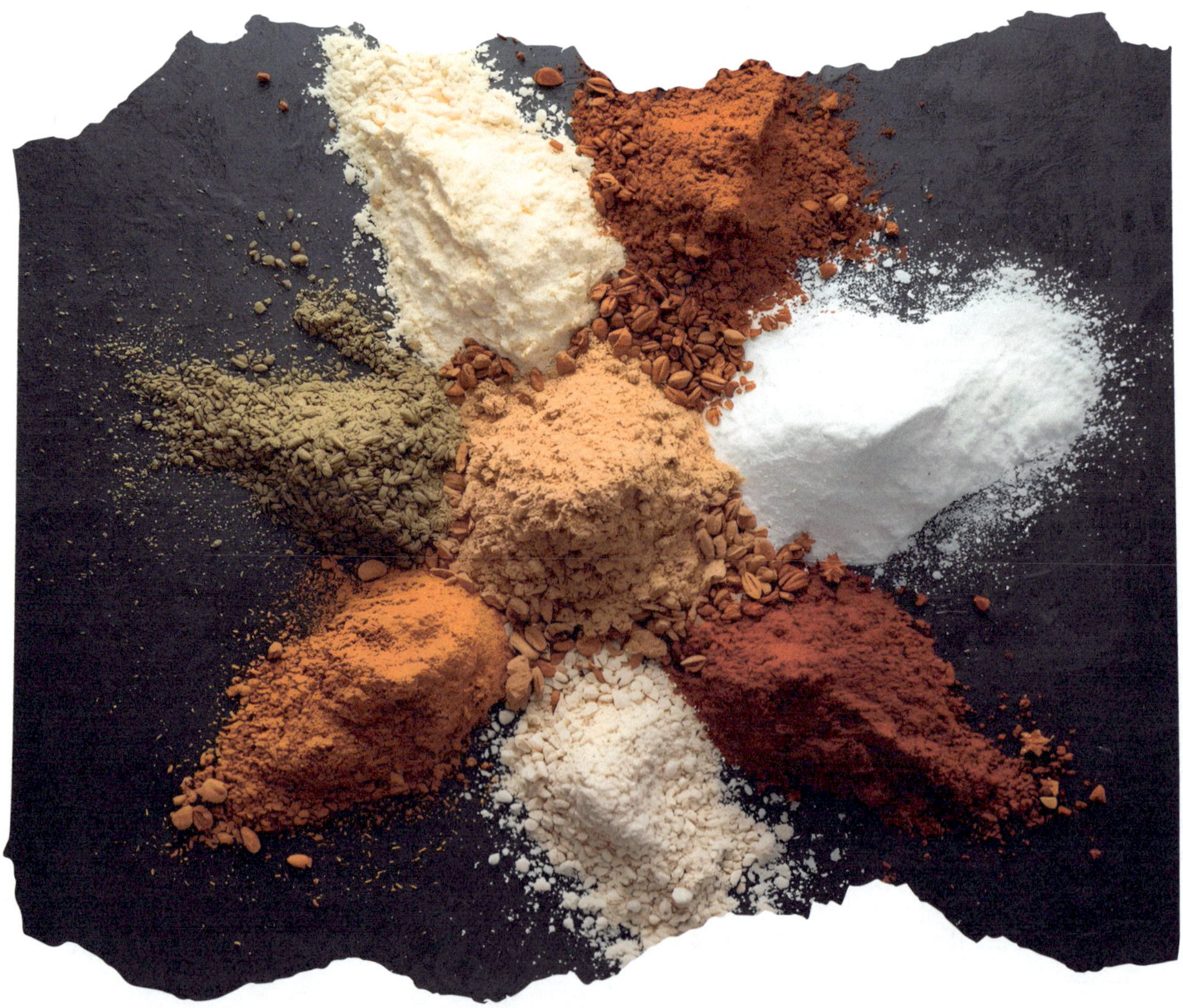

The transition from wheat-based cooking to gluten-free cooking involves much more than simply swapping one flour for another. Gluten is not just an ingredient—it's a natural system that provides structure, elasticity, and moisture retention in traditional baking. It's the reason bread rises high and airy, pasta stretches without tearing, and cakes hold together with a tender crumb. When you remove gluten, those functions don't disappear—they simply need to be replaced by other ingredients working together in new ways.

This is where the real art of gluten-free cooking begins. Instead of thinking in terms of one-for-one substitutions, think in terms of teams: protein-rich flours like almond or chickpea that bring density and nutrition; starch-based flours like rice or tapioca that lighten and lift; and binding agents like xanthan gum or psyllium husk that hold everything together. No single ingredient can mimic gluten's role, but when you understand how to combine them, you can achieve results every bit as satisfying as wheat-based baking—and sometimes even better.

Understanding these ingredient roles transforms you from someone who follows recipes word-for-word into a confident cook who can troubleshoot and adapt along the way. If a cake turns out too dense, you'll recognize it as an imbalance of protein-heavy flours. If bread bakes up gummy, you'll know it's too much starch or binder. Rather than viewing these challenges as failures, you'll see them as valuable clues that guide you toward success the next time.

And gluten-free ingredients go far beyond baking. Flours and starches can thicken sauces, coat proteins for crisp frying, or transform into pasta and dumplings that rival their traditional counterparts. Each flour has its own personality—coconut flour's thirst for liquid, almond flour's tender richness, oat flour's hearty sweetness—and learning how to match the right flour to the right job is one of the most empowering skills you can gain in the kitchen.

Equally important is learning how to store and manage your pantry wisely. Because many gluten-free flours are less processed and higher in natural oils, freshness matters more than ever. A spoonful of rancid almond flour can ruin an entire batch of cookies, while stale rice flour can leave baked goods gritty. Developing smart storage habits—airtight containers, proper refrigeration or freezing, clear labeling—protects your investment and ensures that every recipe starts with the best possible ingredients.

Gluten-free cooking is as much about technique and understanding as it is about the ingredients themselves. Mastering these flours, starches, and binders is like learning a new language: at first it feels unfamiliar, but over time you'll gain fluency, instinct, and creativity. This chapter will walk you through the science, the strategies, and the small adjustments that make the biggest difference—so you can stop worrying about what you've given up and start celebrating what's possible in your gluten-free kitchen.

The Science Behind Gluten-Free Substitutions

The transition from wheat-based cooking to gluten-free cooking involves more than simply swapping one flour for another. Gluten is more than an ingredient—it's a system. When flour mixes with water, gluten proteins (gliadin and glutenin) link together to form a stretchy network. That network traps gas bubbles from yeast or chemical leaveners, creating the lift, chew, and structure we expect in bread, pizza dough, and even cakes. Gluten also helps dough hold moisture, which keeps baked goods tender and prevents them from crumbling.

In gluten-free cooking, we don't have this natural network—so we recreate it through a team approach. No single ingredient can do what gluten does on its own, but when protein-rich flours, starches, and binding agents work together, they mimic those roles in a way that produces satisfying results. Understanding this teamwork is the key to moving beyond simply following recipes and toward cooking with confidence and flexibility.

Protein-Rich Flours

Almond flour, coconut flour, chickpea flour, and other high-protein bases add structure, density, and nutritional heft to gluten-free recipes. Almond flour is especially popular because it creates moist, tender crumbs and delivers a subtle sweetness, but it can make baked goods heavy if not balanced with lighter starches. Coconut flour is uniquely challenging—it's so absorbent that it pulls in up to six times its weight in liquid. That's why coconut flour recipes often call for extra eggs, additional milk, or fruit purées to keep batters workable. Chickpea flour brings a nutty, savory flavor along with impressive protein, making it an excellent choice for flatbreads, crackers, and savory bakes. These flours are the "muscles" of gluten-free baking: strong, sturdy, and dense.

Starch-Based Flours

To balance those heavy proteins, starches like brown rice flour, white rice flour, tapioca starch, arrowroot powder, or potato starch act as the "balloons" that lighten and expand baked goods. Brown rice flour is the backbone of most all-purpose gluten-free flour blends—it has a neutral flavor and a consistency that plays well with almost everything. Tapioca starch, by contrast, brings chewiness and elasticity; it's what gives gluten-free breads that pleasant stretch. However, too much tapioca or arrowroot can backfire, leading to gummy textures. Think of starches as the scaffolding: they give lift and softness, but need the support of protein-rich flours to prevent collapse.

Binding Agents

Without gluten's glue, baked goods tend to fall apart. That's where binders step in. Xanthan gum is the most widely used—it hydrates in liquid to form a gel that holds everything together and stretches slightly as dough rises. The right amount varies by recipe: a pinch for cookies, a bit more for cakes, and a full teaspoon per cup of flour for yeast breads. Think of it as insurance for your baking efforts—too little and your muffins crumble on contact, too much and you'll create a gummy, unpleasant texture that no amount of frosting can disguise.

Psyllium husk powder is another powerful tool, especially for breads. It forms a gel that not only binds ingredients but also adds chewiness and fiber, creating loaves that look and taste closer to wheat bread. When working with psyllium, expect your dough to feel different than traditional bread dough—it will be slightly more elastic and may even develop a faint purple tint, which is completely normal and bakes out beautifully. For those managing both celiac and diabetes, the added fiber bonus from psyllium is particularly valuable, as it helps moderate blood sugar response.

Ground flaxseed and chia seeds mixed with water can serve as natural, whole-food binders that also add nutrition. To use them effectively, combine one tablespoon of ground flaxseed or chia seeds with three tablespoons of water, let the mixture sit for five minutes until it becomes gel-like, then incorporate it into your recipe as you would an egg. These work especially well in heartier baked goods like muffins, quick breads, and cookies where their slightly nutty flavor complements rather than competes with other ingredients.

Unflavored gelatin, both powdered and sheet varieties, serves as an often-overlooked binding agent that works beautifully in more delicate applications. A small amount dissolved in warm water can improve the texture of gluten-free cakes and help stabilize frostings and mousses. I've found it particularly useful when adapting celebration recipes where presentation matters as much as taste.

Each of these agents has a distinct personality, and learning when to use them is one of the biggest steps in mastering gluten-free baking. Don't be discouraged if your first few attempts require adjustment—even experienced gluten-free bakers keep notes about which binders work best for their favorite recipes.

Why Balance Matters
Protein-rich flours alone can create baked goods that are dense and dry; starches alone result in products that are pale and crumbly. Binding agents without the right balance of flours can make doughs sticky or gummy. But when all three categories work in harmony, you achieve baked goods that rise, hold their shape, stay moist, and taste every bit as satisfying as their wheat-based counterparts.

The interplay between these ingredients becomes even more critical when you're managing blood sugar concerns alongside celiac disease. Protein-rich flours like almond and coconut flour naturally have a lower glycemic impact than starches, but they can't carry a recipe alone without creating unpleasantly heavy results. Strategic use of small amounts of starch-based flours provides the lightness we crave while keeping overall glycemic load reasonable. This is where measuring accurately and following tested recipes becomes your best friend—at least until you develop the intuition to adjust on your own.

Think of gluten-free baking as architecture: the protein-rich flours are the solid bricks, the starches are the light beams and windows, and the binding agents are the mortar that keeps the whole structure intact. Understanding this science allows you to not only follow recipes but also troubleshoot problems (too dry, too gummy, too crumbly) and even invent your own creations with confidence.

Common Binding Pitfalls and Solutions
After years of experimentation in my own kitchen, I've learned that most binding failures fall into predictable patterns. Crumbly results that fall apart at first bite usually signal insufficient binding—try increasing your xanthan gum by 1/4 teaspoon or adding an extra egg. Gummy, sticky textures that cling to the roof of your mouth indicate too much binding agent or insufficient flour—scale back the xanthan gum or psyllium and increase your starch component slightly.

Dense, heavy results often mean you've over-relied on binding agents to compensate for other structural issues. Instead, look at your overall flour blend—you may need more light starches to balance protein-rich flours. And remember that gluten-free batters and doughs benefit enormously from resting time. Let your mixture sit for 10-15 minutes before baking to allow binding agents to fully hydrate and do their work. This simple step has saved countless batches from mediocrity in my kitchen.

Understanding these fundamentals transforms you from someone who nervously follows recipes word-for-word to a confident baker who can adapt, troubleshoot, and create with genuine freedom. That's the real gift of mastering gluten-free binding—not just better baked goods, but the knowledge that dietary restrictions haven't diminished your capabilities one bit.

Beyond Baking: Gluten-Free Thickening and Coating

Gluten-free flours aren't limited to baking—they're powerful tools for improving sauces, soups, and crispy coatings as well. Mastering how to use them beyond the mixing bowl can elevate everyday meals into satisfying, restaurant-quality dishes.

Thickening Soups and Sauces

One of the most common uses for flour in traditional cooking is to thicken liquids, whether in a gravy, cream sauce, or hearty stew. Without wheat flour, gluten-free cooks have several reliable alternatives:

- Tapioca Starch – Known for producing glossy, almost translucent finishes, tapioca starch works beautifully in fruit sauces, gravies, and Asian-style soups. It thickens quickly and creates a smooth texture, but too much can lead to a slightly stretchy or gummy result. Always mix it with cold water or broth before whisking into hot liquids to avoid clumping.
- Arrowroot Powder – A close cousin to tapioca, arrowroot provides similar clear, glossy thickening but with a slightly lighter, silkier finish. It's especially useful in delicate sauces where flavor clarity matters, such as lemon curd or light pan sauces. Like tapioca, it should always be slurried with cold liquid before adding to heat.
- Rice Flour – A more traditional thickener, rice flour adds body and opacity, making it ideal for cream-based sauces and chowders. While it can sometimes create a faintly grainy texture if undercooked, simmering the sauce an extra few minutes usually solves the problem. It's also less likely to become gummy than tapioca.
- Almond Flour or Pureed Vegetables – For a nutrient-dense option, almond flour or vegetable purées (like cauliflower or carrots) can be blended in for body and richness. These not only thicken but also enhance nutrition and flavor, making them excellent choices for health-conscious comfort food.

Tips for Success:

Add starch-based thickeners near the end of cooking; prolonged boiling can thin them back out.

For cream sauces, use rice flour or a mix of rice flour and arrowroot to balance creaminess with silkiness.

Always whisk thoroughly to prevent lumps, and avoid adding starches directly to boiling liquid.

Coating and Breading

Without wheat flour or breadcrumbs, gluten-free coatings require a little creativity—but the results can be every bit as crunchy and flavorful, sometimes even more so.

- Almond Flour + Tapioca Starch – This combination delivers a crisp, golden crust that holds up well to baking or frying. The almond flour provides richness and nutty flavor, while tapioca starch ensures the coating adheres tightly and crisps beautifully. It's perfect for chicken tenders, fish fillets, or vegetable fritters.
- Gluten-Free Oat Flour or Rolled Oats – Finely ground oats create a hearty, bread-like coating that's especially good for oven-baked dishes or rustic recipes like meatloaf topping. Whole rolled oats can even be pulsed lightly for a chunkier, crunchier crust.
- Coconut Flour – Coconut flour makes an ultra-crispy, light coating but browns faster than other flours. It's best for shallow frying or recipes where a golden crust develops quickly, like shrimp or zucchini sticks. Keep heat moderate to avoid burning.
- Chickpea Flour – For savory or spiced applications, chickpea flour creates a sturdy coating that pairs well with Mediterranean or Indian flavors. It's slightly denser but holds up to frying and adds plant-based protein to the dish.

Tips for Success:

Use the classic three-step breading method (dip in seasoned flour, then egg wash, then final coating) for the best adherence.
Season your coating well—gluten-free flours tend to be neutral, so salt, pepper, herbs, and spices make a big difference.

For oven-baked coatings, mist lightly with oil spray to encourage browning and crispness without deep frying.

Mix and match coatings to customize texture: for example, almond flour for richness + coconut flour for crispness = a lighter, crunchier crust.

Quick Reference Pairing Guide: Gluten-Free Thickeners & Coatings

For Thickening Soups & Sauces

Creamy Sauces & Chowders → Rice Flour (smooth, opaque finish)

Clear, Glossy Sauces → Arrowroot Powder (light, silky texture)

Fruit Sauces & Gravies → Tapioca Starch (glossy, rich body)

Nutrient-Dense Soups → Almond Flour or Pureed Vegetables (added flavor & fiber)

For Coating & Breading

Crispy, Golden Cutlets or Fish → Almond Flour + Tapioca Starch (balanced crunch & flavor)

Rustic or Oven-Baked Dishes → Gluten-Free Oat Flour or Rolled Oats (hearty, bread-like coating)

Ultra-Crisp, Quick Frying → Coconut Flour (light crunch, browns fast)

Savory, Protein-Rich Coating → Chickpea Flour (earthy flavor, sturdy crust)

Tips at a Glance

Mix starch with cold liquid first → prevents lumps in sauces.

Use three-step breading (flour → egg → coating) → ensures even, lasting crusts.

Mist oven-baked coatings with oil → helps achieve that golden, fried look without deep frying.

Storage and Freshness Tips

One of the hidden challenges of gluten-free cooking is ingredient freshness. Unlike traditional wheat flour, which is highly refined and relatively shelf-stable, many gluten-free flours are minimally processed and retain more of their natural oils. This makes them nutritionally rich but also more perishable. A well-managed storage system will help protect both your investment and your results in the kitchen.

Nut- and Seed-Based Flours

Almond flour, coconut flour, flaxseed meal, and sunflower seed flour all contain natural oils that can turn rancid quickly if exposed to heat, light, or air. Always store these in airtight containers in the refrigerator or freezer. Freezing doesn't affect their performance in recipes, so don't hesitate to keep larger bags in the freezer and refill a small jar for daily use. Expect a shelf life of about 3–6 months in the fridge and up to a year in the freezer.

Grain-Based Flours

Brown rice flour, sorghum flour, millet flour, and buckwheat flour also contain oils, but at lower levels. These can be safely stored in airtight containers at room temperature for a few months, but refrigeration is still the safer bet if you live in a warm or humid climate. White rice flour is the exception—it's more processed and has a longer room-temperature shelf life, though it still benefits from airtight storage.

Starches

Tapioca starch, arrowroot powder, and potato starch are low in oils and generally more stable. These can be stored in a cool, dry pantry for 6–12 months. Just be sure they're kept in airtight containers to prevent clumping from humidity.

Labeling & Rotation

Because gluten-free flours don't always have obvious expiration dates printed on resealable bags, it's wise to label each container with the purchase date. Try to rotate your flours so the oldest gets used first. A simple masking tape label or chalk marker on jars goes a long way toward keeping your system organized.

How to Check Freshness

- Smell: Rancid nut or seed flours will smell bitter, soapy, or metallic instead of fresh and nutty. If it smells "off," toss it.
- Texture: Starches and rice flours should be light and powdery. If they feel clumpy, damp, or gritty, humidity may have compromised them.
- Taste: A small pinch should taste neutral or mildly nutty. Any bitter aftertaste is a sign of spoilage.

Troubleshooting with Old Flours

Sometimes you don't realize a flour has gone stale until your recipe doesn't turn out. Here are common problems linked to flour freshness:

- Unexpected Bitterness in Baked Goods → Likely rancid nut flour. Solution: discard and replace; always store in fridge/freezer.
- Clumpy or Gummy Sauces → Starch has absorbed moisture. Solution: sift flour before use; store in airtight jars with silica packs if humidity is high.
- Flat or Dense Results → Old flours lose some of their ability to absorb liquid properly. Solution: replace with a fresher batch; store smaller amounts at a time.

Buying Smarter

Until you know which flours you'll use most, buy in smaller amounts. Specialty flours can be expensive, and it's frustrating to throw out half a bag. Many health food stores and co-ops sell gluten-free flours in bulk bins, allowing you to experiment with a cup or two at a time. Once you find your favorites, consider buying larger bags online for better pricing, then dividing them into smaller airtight containers for storage.

The Big Picture

Treat gluten-free flours as living ingredients, not pantry fillers. Their freshness directly affects the taste and texture of your food. A simple storage system—airtight jars, cool storage, careful labeling—will not only extend their shelf life but also improve your confidence as a gluten-free cook. With practice, you'll learn the subtle differences between fresh and stale ingredients, and your results will show it.

Sweetener Conversion Chart

Sweetener	Conversion to 1 Cup Sugar	Notes
Stevia (Pure powder or liquid)	1/2 to 1 tsp	Extremely concentrated; blends vary; adjust carefully
Monk Fruit Sweetener	1 tsp to 1 tbsp	Depends on blend; some are cup-for-cup with erythritol
Erythritol	1 cup	Measures like sugar; may cause cooling effect
Allulose	1 cup	Cup-for-cup; browns and caramelizes well
Xylitol	1 cup	Cup-for-cup; toxic to dogs; may upset digestion
Unsweetened Applesauce	1/2 cup	Replace 1 cup sugar with 1/2 cup; reduce liquid
Pure Maple Syrup	3/4 cup	Reduce other liquids by 3 tbsp
Honey	2/3 cup	Natural choice, but need to compensate for liquid
Coconut Sugar	1 Cup	Cup-for-cup; lower glycemic than white sugar
Date Sugar or Paste	2/3 to 1 cup	Adds fiber & flavor; best in dense bakes

Gluten Free Baking Troubleshooting Guide

Problem	Likely Cause	Quick Fix
Too Dry / Crumbly	Not enough binding agent; flour blend too heavy on protein flours; overbaking.	Add more xanthan gum or psyllium (start with ¼ tsp per cup of flour); include an extra egg yolk; fold in moisture-rich ingredients like applesauce, yogurt, or mashed banana; shorten baking time slightly.
Dense / Heavy Texture	Too much almond, coconut, or chickpea flour; not enough leavening.	Replace some protein-rich flour with lighter flours or starches (brown rice, tapioca, or arrowroot); add ¼ tsp extra baking powder per cup of flour.
Gummy or Sticky Center	Overuse of starches (especially tapioca); too much xanthan gum or psyllium; underbaking.	Reduce tapioca or gum by 25–50%; bake a little longer at a slightly lower temperature; measure starches precisely.
Flat / Didn't Rise	Not enough leavening; batter too wet; oven too cool.	Increase baking powder or baking soda slightly; check oven temperature with a thermometer; let batter rest 10–15 minutes before baking so flours and gums hydrate fully.
Falls Apart After Baking	Too little binder; flour blend too light; lack of eggs in recipe.	Increase xanthan gum/psyllium; add a flax or chia "egg" (1 tbsp ground seed + 3 tbsp water = 1 egg); include 1–2 extra eggs if recipe allows.
Overly Sweet or Off Flavor	Strong taste from bean flours; too much coconut flour or stevia.	Blend bean flours with milder flours (rice, oat, almond); reduce coconut flour to 10–15% of total flour; balance flavors with vanilla, cinnamon, or citrus zest.
Stale Quickly	Lack of gluten means moisture escapes faster.	Store baked goods in airtight containers; freeze extras right after cooling; add a tablespoon of honey or glycerin to batter for longer moisture retention.

Icon Definitions

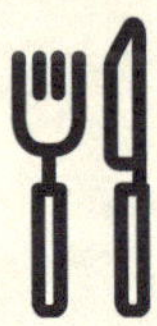

Servings

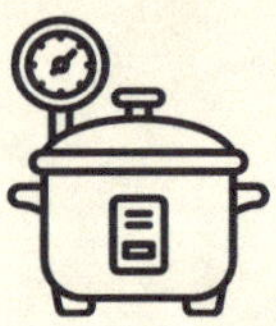

Pressure Cook TIme

Preparation Time

Cook Time

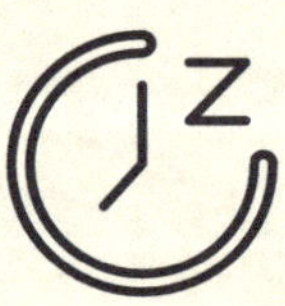

Rest Time

CHAPTER 03

Energizing Breakfasts

These are your everyday breakfast heroes – the recipes you'll turn to on busy weekday mornings when you need something that's both nutritious and realistic. Each recipe is designed to provide sustained energy through a balance of protein, healthy fats and complex carbohydrates, while keeping preparation time reasonable for real-world schedules. Most can be on the table in 15 minutes or less, and several offer make-ahead components to streamline your morning routine even further.

List of Recipes

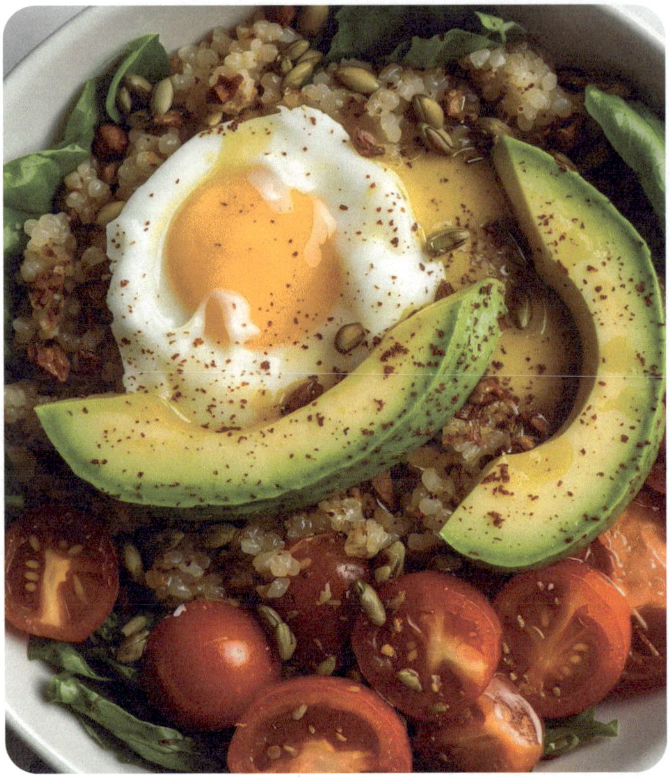

Savory Breakfast Quinoa Bowl

Transform quinoa from a dinner side dish into a protein-packed breakfast base. This savory bowl provides complete protein and can be customized with whatever vegetables you have on hand.

4 | 15 minutes | 1 hour

NUTRITION

Per serving: 385 calories, 17g protein, 34g carbohydrates, 22g fat, 8g fiber

INGREDIENTS

- 1 cup quinoa, rinsed
- 2 cups low-sodium vegetable broth
- 2 tablespoons olive oil
- 4 large eggs
- 2 cups fresh spinach
- 1 medium avocado, sliced
- 1/2 cup cherry tomatoes, halved
- 1/4 cup pumpkin seeds
- 2 tablespoons lemon juice
- Salt and pepper to taste
- Red pepper flakes (optional)

DIRECTIONS

1. In a medium saucepan, bring vegetable broth to a boil. Add quinoa, reduce heat to low, cover and simmer for 15 minutes until liquid is absorbed.
2. Meanwhile, heat 1 tablespoon olive oil in a large skillet over medium heat. Add spinach and cook until wilted, about 2 minutes. Season with salt and pepper.
3. In the same skillet, push spinach to the side and fry eggs to your preference (sunny-side up or over-easy work well).
4. Fluff quinoa with a fork and divide among 4 bowls.
5. Top each bowl with wilted spinach, a fried egg, avocado slices, cherry tomatoes, and pumpkin seeds.
6. Drizzle with remaining olive oil and lemon juice. Season with salt, pepper, and red pepper flakes if desired.

Almond Flour Pancakes

These fluffy, protein-rich pancakes prove that gluten-free doesn't mean flavor-free. Made with almond flour, they're naturally lower in carbohydrates than traditional pancakes while providing healthy fats and protein.

4 (makes 12 pancakes) | 10 minutes | 15 minutes

INGREDIENTS

- 2 cups almond flour
- 6 large eggs
- 1/4 cup unsweetened almond milk
- 2 tablespoons allulose (or sweetener of choice)
- 1 teaspoon vanilla extract
- 1 teaspoon baking powder
- 1/2 teaspoon salt
- 1/4 teaspoon cinnamon
- Coconut oil or butter for cooking

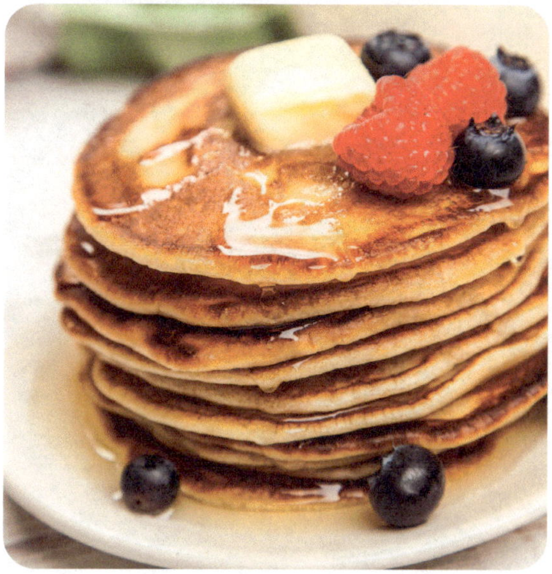

DIRECTIONS

1. In a large bowl, whisk together almond flour, erythritol, baking powder, salt, and cinnamon.
2. In another bowl, beat eggs, then whisk in almond milk and vanilla extract.
3. Pour wet ingredients into dry ingredients and stir until just combined. Let batter rest for 5 minutes to thicken.
4. Heat a large skillet or griddle over medium-low heat. Add a small amount of coconut oil.
5. Pour 1/4 cup batter per pancake onto hot surface. Cook for 2-3 minutes until bubbles form on surface and edges look set.
6. Flip carefully and cook for 1-2 minutes more until golden brown.
7. Serve immediately or keep warm in 200°F oven.

NUTRITION

Per serving, 3 pancakes: 320 calories, 18g protein, 10g carbohydrates, 25g fat, 5g fiber

Smoked Salmon Cucumber Boats

2	10 minutes	0 minutes

An elegant, low-carb breakfast that feels special enough for weekend entertaining but simple enough for busy mornings. The healthy fats from salmon and avocado provide lasting satiety.

DIRECTIONS

1. Cut cucumbers in half lengthwise. Using a spoon, scoop out seeds and some flesh to create boats.
2. In a small bowl, mix mashed avocado, cream cheese, chopped dill, and lemon juice until smooth.
3. Spread avocado mixture evenly in cucumber boats.
4. Top with pieces of smoked salmon and capers.
5. Season with black pepper and garnish with fresh dill sprigs.
6. Serve immediately.

INGREDIENTS

- 2 large cucumbers
- 4 oz smoked salmon, torn into pieces
- 1/2 ripe avocado, mashed
- 2 tablespoons cream cheese, softened
- 1 tablespoon fresh dill, chopped
- 1 tablespoon capers
- 1 tablespoon lemon juice
- Black pepper to taste
- Fresh dill sprigs for garnish

NUTRITION

Per serving: 245 calories, 18g protein, 8g carbohydrates, 16g fat, 4g fiber

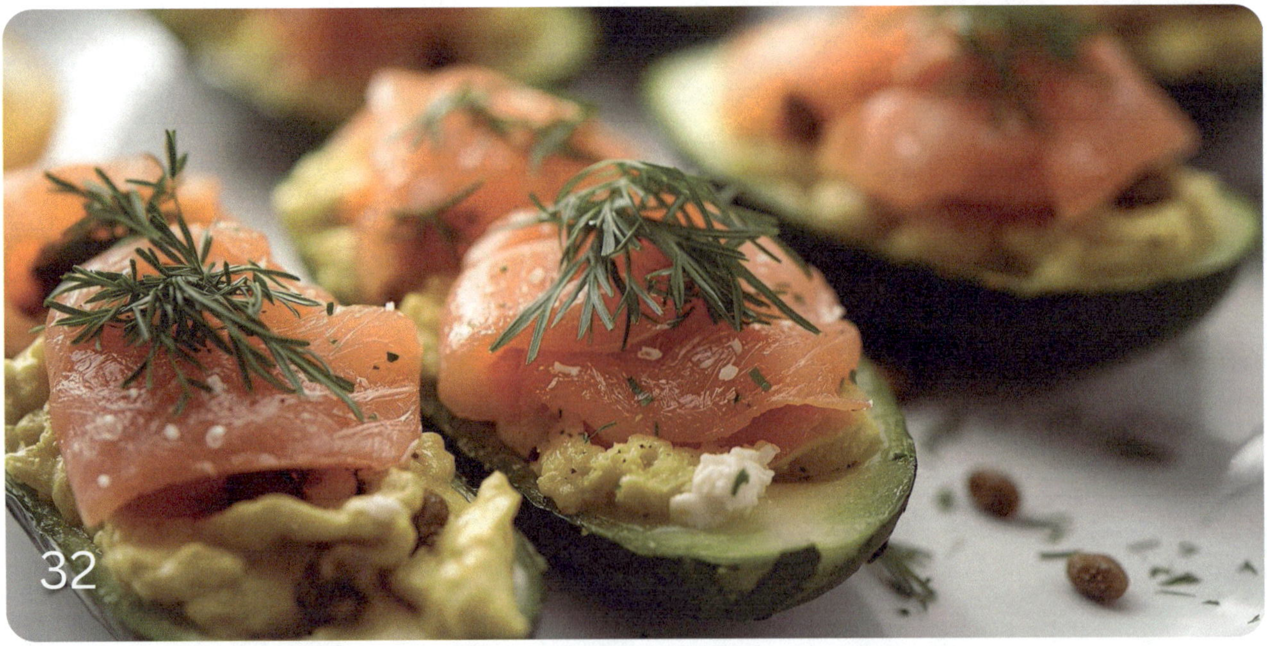

Greek Yogurt Berry Bowl

Servings	Prep time	Cook time
1	3 minutes	0 minutes

A simple but satisfying breakfast that combines protein-rich Greek yogurt with antioxidant-packed berries and healthy fats from nuts and seeds.

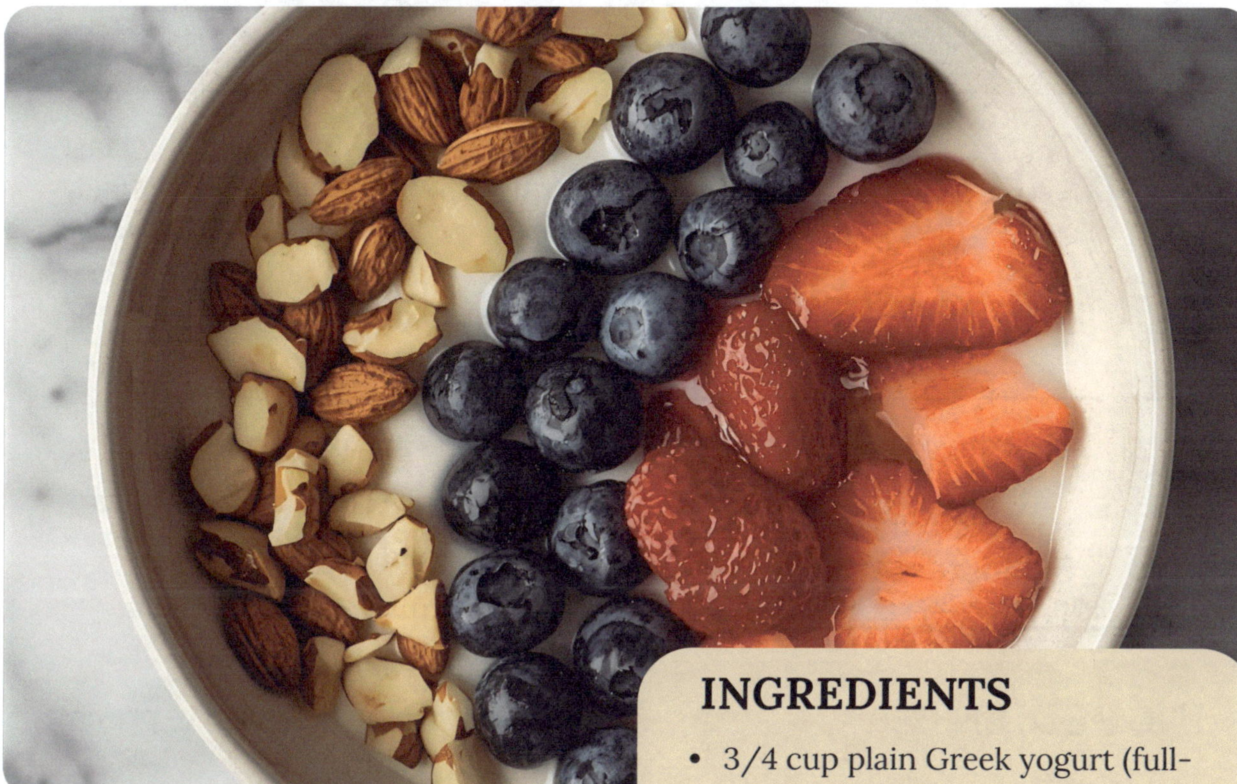

INGREDIENTS

- 3/4 cup plain Greek yogurt (full-fat)
- 1/2 cup mixed fresh berries (blueberries, strawberries, raspberries)
- 2 tablespoons chopped almonds or walnuts
- 1 tablespoon ground flaxseed
- 1 teaspoon honey or sugar free maple syrup (optional)
- 1/4 teaspoon vanilla extract
- Pinch of cinnamon

DIRECTIONS

1. In a bowl, stir vanilla extract and sweetener (if using) into Greek yogurt.
2. Top with fresh berries, nuts, and ground flaxseed.
3. Sprinkle with cinnamon and serve immediately.

NUTRITION

Per serving: 295 calories, 20g protein, 18g carbohydrates, 18g fat, 7g fiber

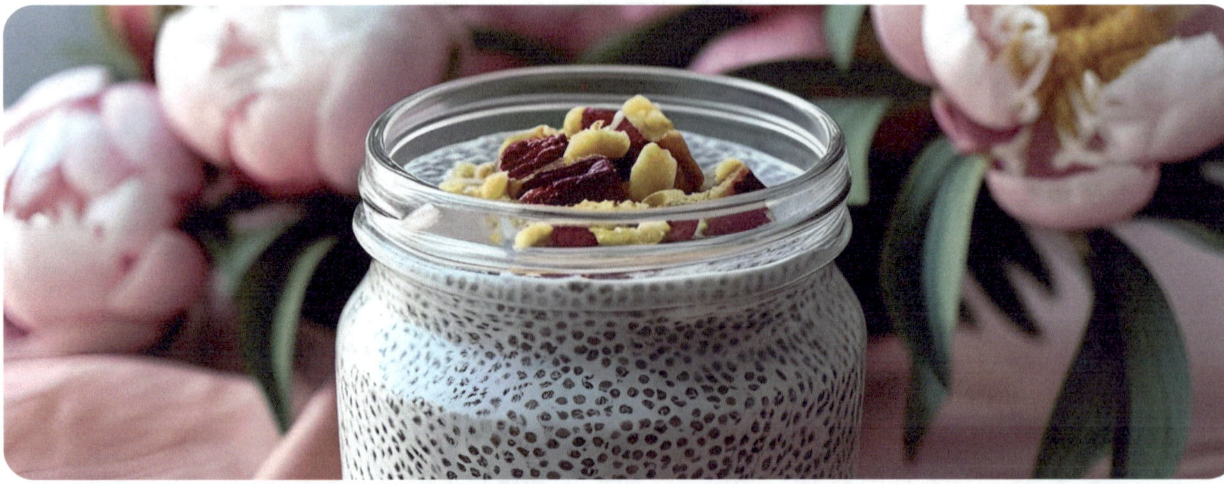

Coconut Chia Pudding

This creamy, pudding-like breakfast requires no cooking and actually improves overnight. Chia seeds provide omega-3 fatty acids, fiber, and plant-based protein.

Servings	Prep time	Cook time
4	5 minutes (plus 4 hour chilling)	0 minutes

INGREDIENTS

- 1/2 cup chia seeds
- 2 cups canned coconut milk (full-fat)
- 2 tablespoons erythritol or maple syrup
- 1 teaspoon vanilla extract
- Pinch of salt
- 1/2 cup fresh berries for serving
- 1/4 cup sliced almonds for serving
- 2 tablespoons unsweetened coconut flakes for serving

DIRECTIONS

1. In a large bowl, whisk together coconut milk, sweetener, vanilla extract, and salt until well combined.
2. Add chia seeds and whisk vigorously for 2 minutes to prevent clumping.
3. Cover and refrigerate for at least 4 hours or overnight, whisking once more after the first hour.
4. Stir pudding before serving. Divide among 4 bowls or jars.
5. Top with fresh berries, sliced almonds, and coconut flakes.

NUTRITION

Per serving: 315 calories, 8g protein, 15g carbohydrates, 26g fat, 12g fiber

Sweet Potato Hash with Eggs

6	15 minutes	25 minutes

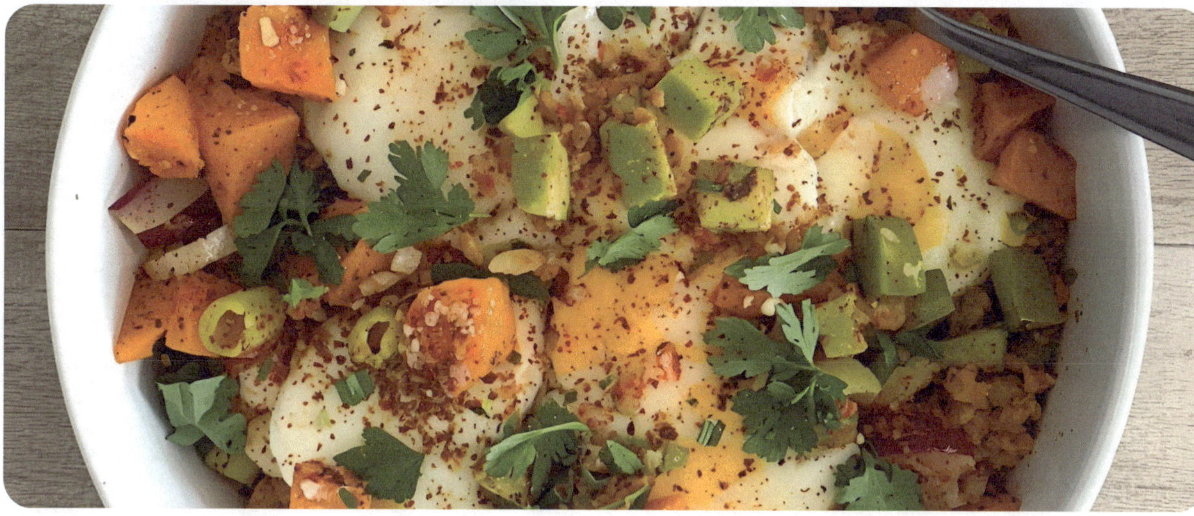

This hearty, one-pan breakfast combines the natural sweetness of roasted sweet potatoes with savory vegetables and protein-rich eggs. It's substantial enough to fuel active mornings.

DIRECTIONS

1. Preheat oven to 425°F (220°C).
2. Toss diced sweet potatoes with 2 tablespoons olive oil, salt, and pepper. Spread on a large baking sheet and roast for 15 minutes.
3. Heat remaining oil in a large oven-safe skillet over medium heat. Add onion and bell pepper, cooking for 5 minutes until softened.
4. Add garlic, paprika, and cumin, cooking for 1 minute until fragrant.
5. Add roasted sweet potatoes to the skillet and stir to combine. Season with salt and pepper.
6. Using a spoon, make 6 wells in the hash. Crack an egg into each well.
7. Transfer skillet to oven and bake for 8-10 minutes until egg whites are set but yolks are still slightly runny.
8. Remove from oven, sprinkle with cilantro, and serve with avocado slices.

INGREDIENTS

- 2 large sweet potatoes, peeled and diced (about 4 cups)
- 3 tablespoons olive oil
- 1 large bell pepper, diced
- 1 medium onion, diced
- 2 cloves garlic, minced
- 6 large eggs
- 1 teaspoon paprika
- 1/2 teaspoon ground cumin
- Salt and black pepper to taste
- 2 tablespoons fresh cilantro, chopped
- 1 avocado, sliced (for serving)

NUTRITION

Per serving: 285 calories, 12g protein, 22g carbohydrates, 17g fat, 4g fiber

Protein-Packed Veggie Scramble

This versatile scramble transforms simple eggs into a complete, satisfying meal. The combination of vegetables adds fiber and nutrients while the generous protein content helps maintain stable blood sugar throughout the morning.

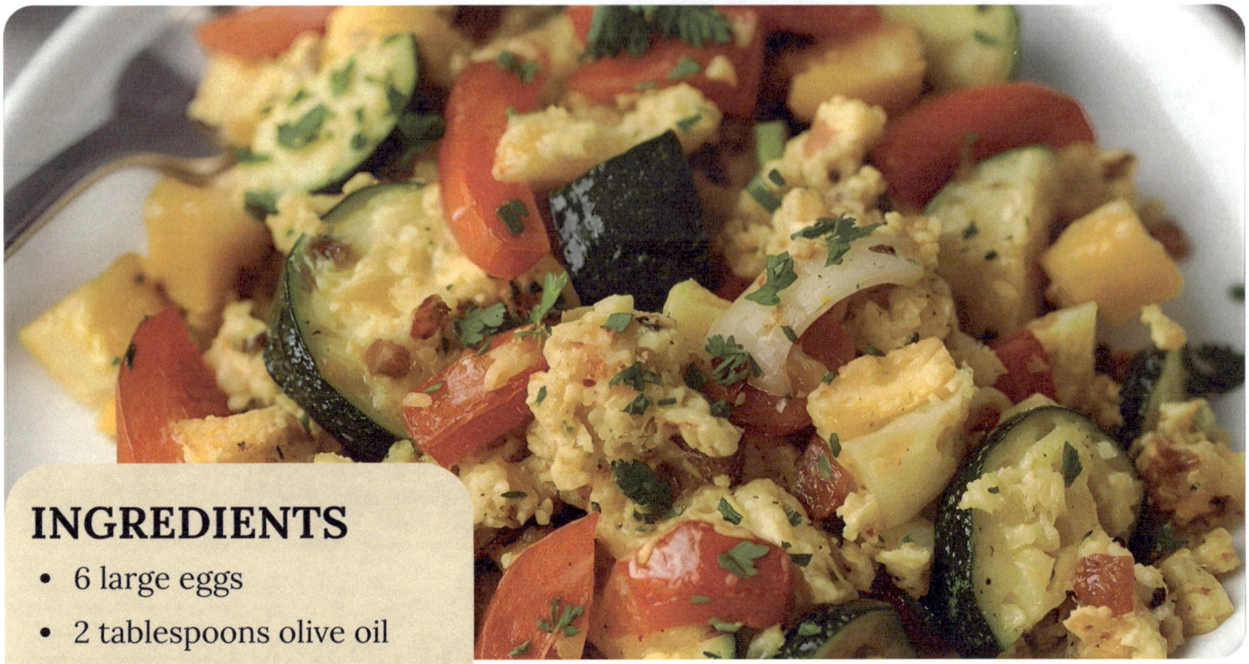

INGREDIENTS

- 6 large eggs
- 2 tablespoons olive oil
- 1 medium bell pepper, diced
- 1 medium zucchini, diced
- 1/2 medium onion, diced
- 2 cloves garlic, minced
- 1/2 teaspoon dried oregano
- Salt and black pepper to taste
- 2 tablespoons fresh parsley, chopped (optional)

NUTRITION

Per serving: 285 calories, 20g protein, 8g carbohydrates, 20g fat, 3g fiber

2 | 8 minutes | 5 minutes

DIRECTIONS

1. Heat olive oil in a large non-stick skillet over medium heat.
2. Add onion and cook for 2 minutes until softened. Add bell pepper and zucchini, cooking for 3-4 minutes until vegetables are tender-crisp.
3. Add garlic and oregano, cooking for 30 seconds until fragrant.
4. Beat eggs in a bowl with salt and pepper. Pour into skillet with vegetables.
5. Using a spatula, gently scramble eggs and vegetables together until eggs are set but still creamy, about 2-3 minutes.
6. Remove from heat, sprinkle with fresh parsley if using, and serve immediately.

Green Smoothie Bowl

Servings	Prep time	Cook time
2	8 minutes	0 minutes

This nutrient-dense smoothie bowl packs vegetables into a sweet, creamy breakfast that tastes like dessert. The frozen banana creates a thick, ice cream-like texture.

INGREDIENTS

For the smoothie base:

- 1 frozen banana
- 1 cup fresh spinach
- 1/2 ripe avocado
- 1 cup unsweetened almond milk
- 1 tablespoon almond butter
- 1 teaspoon vanilla extract
- 1 tablespoon ground flax seed
- 1 cup ice cubes

For toppings:

- 1/4 cup fresh berries
- 2 tablespoons chopped almonds
- 1 tablespoon chia seeds
- 1 tablespoon unsweetened coconut flakes

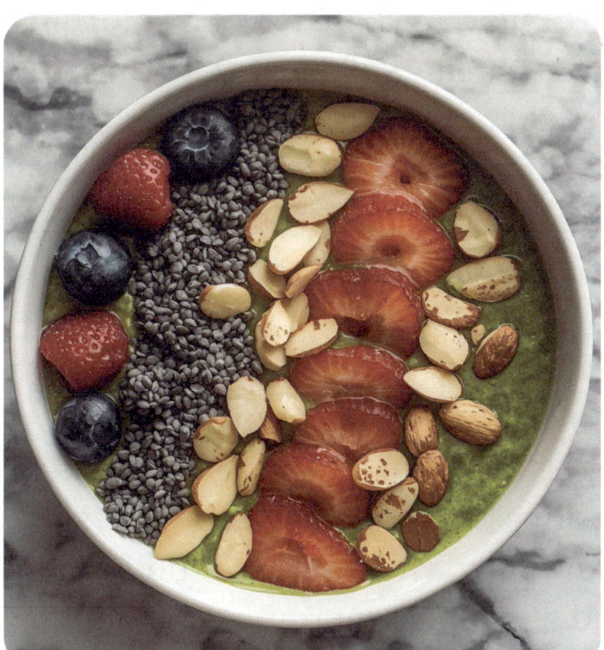

DIRECTIONS

1. Add all smoothie base ingredients to a high-speed blender.
2. Blend on high speed until smooth and creamy, about 1-2 minutes. The mixture should be thick enough to eat with a spoon.
3. Divide between 2 bowls.
4. Arrange toppings over smoothie base in sections for an attractive presentation.
5. Serve immediately with spoons.

NUTRITION

Per serving: 275 calories, 8g protein, 25g carbohydrates, 17g fat, 10g fiber

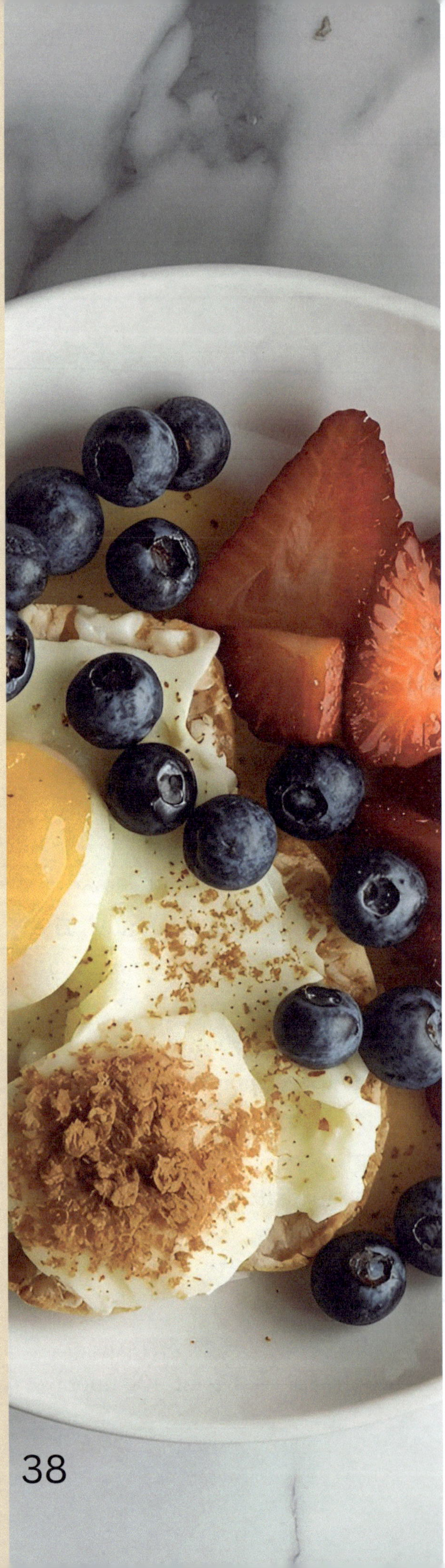

Tips For Success

Prep Vegetables in Advance: Wash, chop, and store vegetables in the refrigerator for up to 3 days. This makes weekday breakfast assembly much faster.

Batch Cook Grains: Cook quinoa or other grains in larger batches over the weekend and refrigerate in portions for easy morning assembly.

Customize to Your Preferences: These recipes are designed to be flexible. Swap vegetables based on what you have available, adjust seasonings to your taste, and modify portions as needed.

Blood Sugar Timing: If you're particularly sensitive to morning blood sugar spikes, try eating the protein and fat components of your breakfast first, then adding any higher-carb ingredients 10-15 minutes later.

Remember, consistency matters more than perfection. Having a repertoire of reliable breakfast options makes it easier to start every day with stable blood sugar and sustained energy.

CHAPTER 04

Make-Ahead Morning Solutions

Busy mornings don't have to derail your commitment to healthy eating. These recipes are designed to transform your most chaotic weekday moments into opportunities for nourishing yourself well. By investing a small amount of time during your weekend prep sessions, you can ensure that even your most rushed mornings include a satisfying, blood sugar-friendly breakfast. Most of these recipes actually improve with time, developing deeper flavors and better textures after sitting overnight or longer.

List of Recipes

1. Smoked Salmon and Spinach Frittata
2. Freezer Breakfast Burritos
3. Breakfast Egg Muffins
4. Overnight Steel Cut Oats
5. Chia Pudding Parfait Cups
6. Super Protein Shake Packs
7. Baked Oatmeal Squares

Smoked Salmon & Spinach Frittata

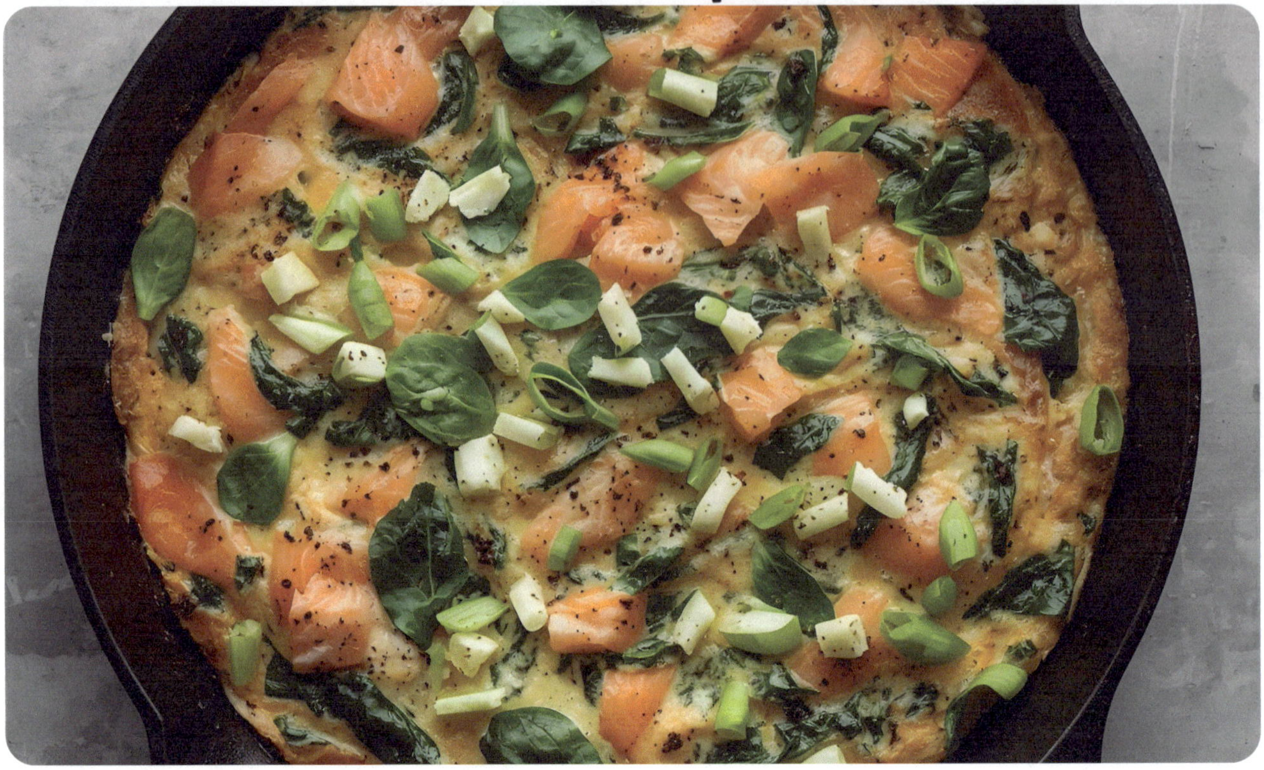

A light, protein-packed frittata with smoked salmon, tender spinach, and creamy goat cheese.

Servings	Prep time	Cook time
6	10 minutes	25 minutes

INGREDIENTS

- 8 large eggs
- ½ cup almond milk
- 4 oz smoked salmon, chopped
- 2 cups baby spinach
- 3 green onions, sliced
- ½ cup crumbled goat cheese (optional)
- Salt and black pepper to taste
- 1 tbsp olive oil

NUTRITION

Per serving without goat cheese: 180 calories, 11g protein, 3g carbohydrates, 13g fat, 1g fiber

STORAGE

Keeps 3 days refrigerated;
Serve warm or cold.

DIRECTIONS

1. Preheat oven to 350°F (175°C).
2. In a bowl, whisk eggs, almond milk, salt, and pepper.
3. Heat oil in an oven-safe skillet; sauté spinach and green onions until wilted.
4. Scatter salmon and goat cheese over vegetables. Pour egg mixture into skillet.
5. Cook undisturbed 2–3 min, then transfer to oven and bake 15–20 min, until set and lightly browned.
6. Cool slightly before slicing.

These protein-packed burritos wrap up a complete breakfast in convenient, freezer-friendly packages perfect for busy mornings.

Freezer Breakfast Burritos

Servings	Prep time	Cook time
8	30 minutes	15 minutes

INGREDIENTS

- 8 large gluten-free tortillas
- 12 large eggs, scrambled
- 2 cups cooked black beans, drained and rinsed
- 2 cups sweet potato, roasted and diced (optional)
- 1 cup shredded cheese
- 1 large bell pepper, diced
- 1 medium onion, diced
- 2 tablespoons olive oil
- 1 teaspoon cumin
- 1 teaspoon paprika
- Salt and pepper to taste
- 1 cup salsa (for serving)

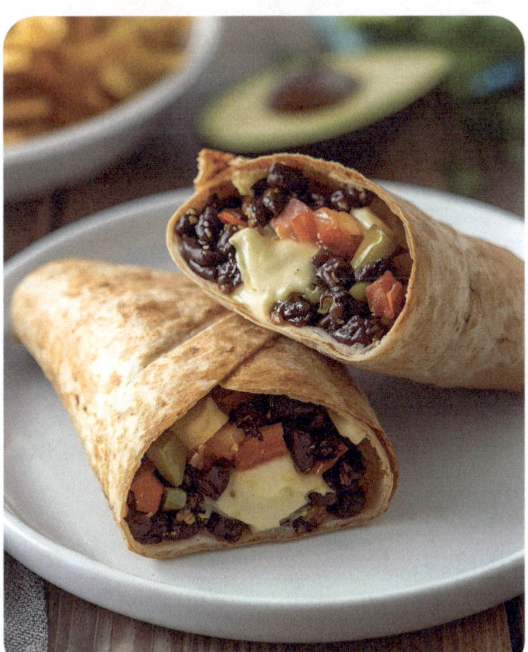

DIRECTIONS

1. Preheat oven to 400°F (200°C). Toss diced sweet potato with 1 tablespoon olive oil, salt, and pepper. Roast for 20 minutes until tender.
2. Heat remaining oil in large skillet over medium heat. Sauté onion and bell pepper for 5 minutes until softened.
3. Add cumin and paprika, cooking for 1 minute until fragrant.
4. Add black beans and roasted sweet potatoes, stirring to combine. Season with salt and pepper.
5. Scramble eggs in a separate pan until just set but still creamy.
6. To assemble: Place 1/8 of egg mixture, bean mixture, and cheese (if using) in center of each tortilla.
7. Fold in sides, then roll tightly from bottom to top.
8. Wrap individually in aluminum foil and freeze.

NUTRITION

Per serving: 385 calories, 18g protein, 45g carbohydrates, 15g fat, 8g fiber

STORAGE

Freeze for up to 3 months. To reheat: Remove foil, wrap in damp paper towel, and microwave for 2-3 minutes, turning halfway through.

Breakfast Egg Muffins

Servings	Prep time	Cook time
6	15 minutes	20 minutes

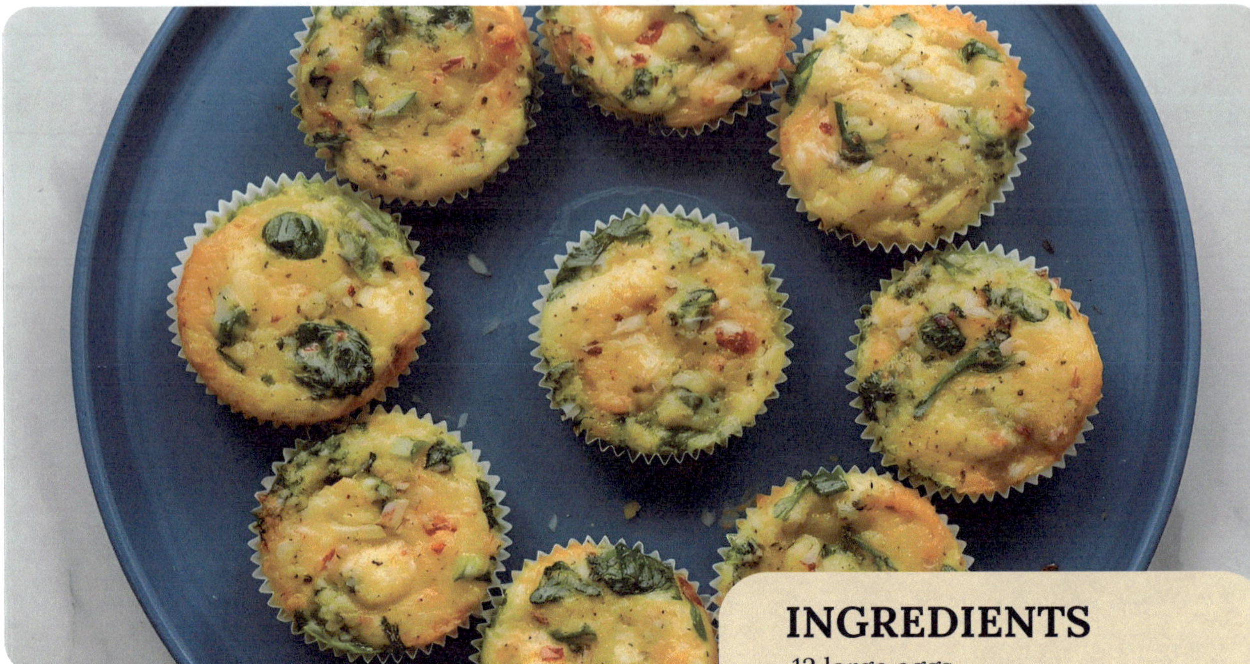

These protein-packed, portable egg muffins can be customized with your favorite vegetables and make perfect grab-and-go breakfasts for the entire week.

INGREDIENTS

- 12 large eggs
- 1/4 cup unsweetened almond milk
- 1 cup fresh spinach, chopped
- 1/2 cup bell pepper, finely diced
- 1/2 cup zucchini, finely diced
- 1/4 cup red onion, finely diced
- 1/2 cup shredded Swiss cheese
- 2 tablespoons olive oil
- 1 teaspoon dried herbs (oregano, thyme, or Italian seasoning)
- Salt and black pepper to taste
- Cooking spray

DIRECTIONS

1. Preheat oven to 350°F (175°C). Spray a 12-cup muffin tin with cooking spray.
2. Heat olive oil in a large skillet over medium heat. Sauté onion, bell pepper, and zucchini for 5 minutes until softened.
3. Add spinach and cook until wilted, about 1 minute. Remove from heat and let cool slightly.
4. In a large bowl, whisk eggs and almond milk until well combined. Season with herbs, salt, and pepper.
5. Divide sautéed vegetables evenly among muffin cups. Pour egg mixture over vegetables, filling each cup about 3/4 full.
6. Sprinkle with cheese if using.
7. Bake for 18-20 minutes until eggs are set and tops are lightly golden.
8. Cool in pan for 5 minutes before removing.

NUTRITION

Per serving, 2 muffins: 215 calories, 16g protein, 4g carbohydrates, 15g fat, 1g fiber

STORAGE

Refrigerate for up to 4 days or freeze for up to 3 months. Reheat from frozen in microwave for 1-2 minutes.

Overnight Steel-Cut Oats

Servings	Prep time	Cook time
6	10 minutes	8 hours (slow cooker)

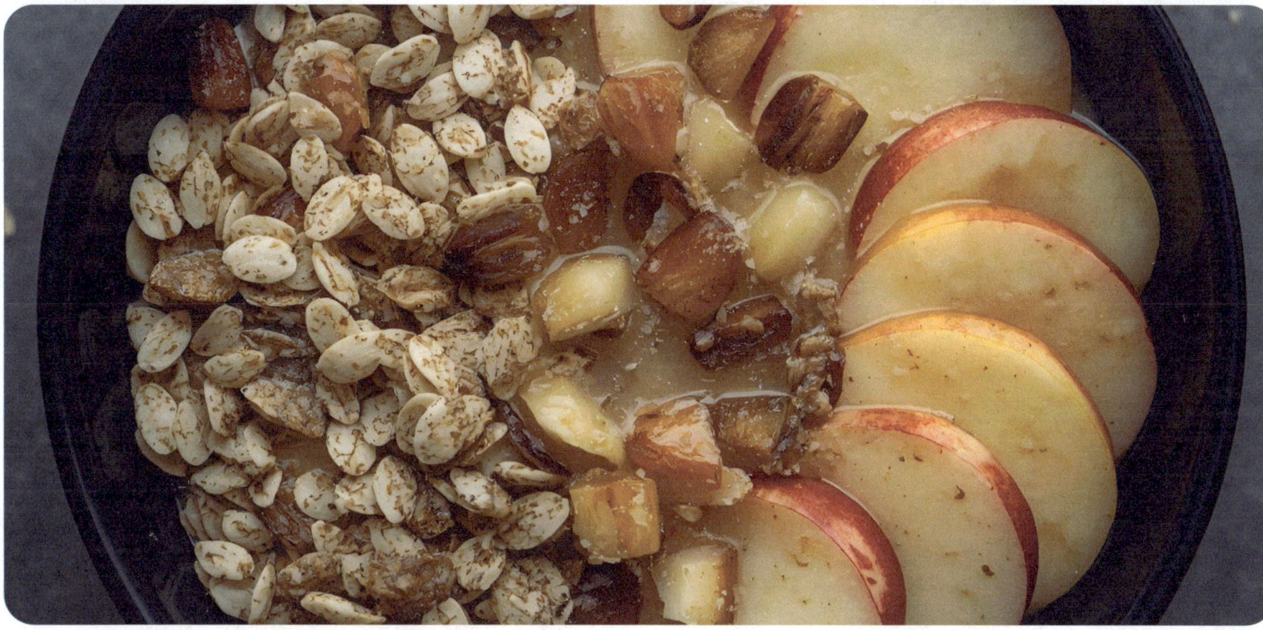

INGREDIENTS

- 1 cup steel-cut oats (certified gluten-free)
- 4 cups water
- 1 cup unsweetened almond milk
- 2 medium apples, peeled and diced
- 1/4 cup chopped walnuts
- 2 tablespoons ground flaxseed
- 1 teaspoon cinnamon
- 1/2 teaspoon vanilla extract
- 1/4 teaspoon salt
- 2 tablespoons sugar free maple syrup (optional)

Transform steel-cut oats into a creamy, ready-to-eat breakfast using your slow cooker. This hands-off method creates perfectly tender oats with minimal morning effort.

DIRECTIONS

1. Spray slow cooker with cooking spray or lightly grease.
2. Combine all ingredients in slow cooker and stir well.
3. Cook on low for 8 hours or overnight.
4. Stir before serving. Add additional almond milk if thinner consistency is desired.
5. Serve warm, or refrigerate portions for up to 5 days.
6. To reheat: Add splash of milk and microwave for 1-2 minutes, stirring halfway through.

NUTRITION

Per serving: 195 calories, 6g protein, 32g carbohydrates, 6g fat, 6g fiber

STORAGE

Refrigerate in individual portions for up to 5 days. Freezes for up to 3 months.

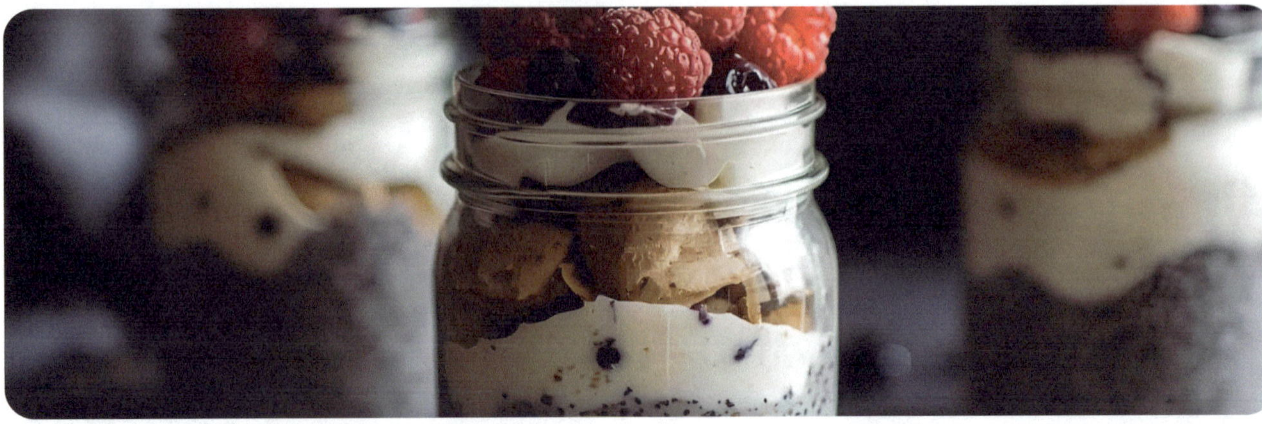

Chia Pudding Parfait Jars

Servings	Prep time	Cook time
4	15 minutes (plus 4 hours chilling)	0 minutes

INGREDIENTS

For chia pudding:

- 1/2 cup chia seeds
- 2 cups unsweetened coconut milk (canned)
- 3 tablespoons allulose or sugar free maple syrup
- 1 teaspoon vanilla extract
- Pinch of salt

For layers:

- 2 cups mixed fresh berries
- 1/2 cup chopped almonds
- 1/4 cup unsweetened coconut flakes
- 2 tablespoons ground flax seed

Layer nutrient-dense chia pudding with fresh berries for a beautiful, Instagram-worthy breakfast that's ready when you are.

DIRECTIONS

1. In a large bowl, whisk together coconut milk, sweetener, vanilla, and salt.
2. Add chia seeds and whisk vigorously for 2 minutes to prevent clumping.
3. Cover and refrigerate for at least 4 hours or overnight, whisking once after the first hour.
4. To assemble parfaits: In 4 mason jars or glasses, layer 1/4 of the chia pudding, followed by berries, nuts, and coconut flakes.
5. Repeat layers, ending with a sprinkle of flaxseed on top.
6. Seal and refrigerate until ready to eat.

NUTRITION

Per serving: 355 calories, 10g protein, 20g carbohydrates, 28g fat, 15g fiber

STORAGE

Assembled parfaits keep for up to 3 days in refrigerator.

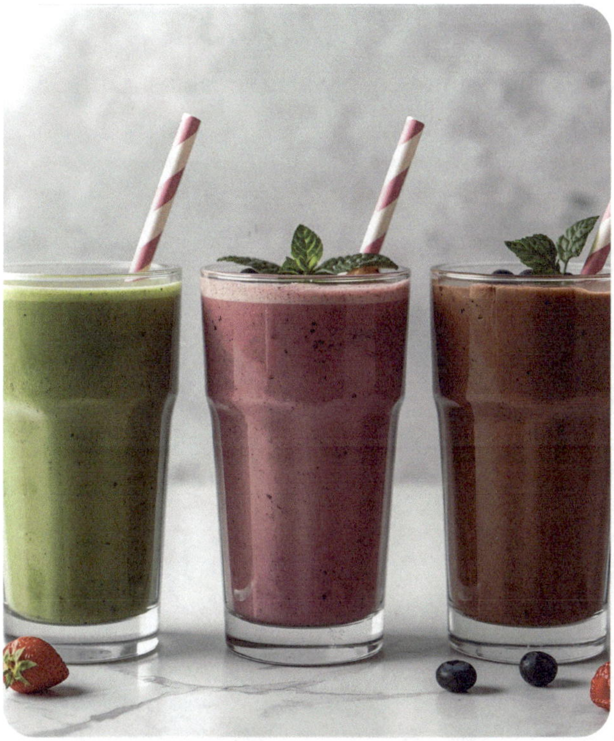

Super Protein Smoothie Packs

Pre-portioned smoothie ingredients that transform into nutritious breakfasts with just the addition of liquid and 60 seconds in the blender.

Servings	Prep time	Cook time
8	20 minutes	0 minutes

NUTRITION

Per serving per smoothie: 245 calories, 8g protein, 28g carbohydrates, 12g fat, 8g fiber

STORAGE

Frozen packs keep for up to 3 months.

INGREDIENTS

Green Goddess Pack (makes 2 packs):

- 2 cups fresh spinach
- 1 frozen banana, sliced
- 1/2 avocado, cubed
- 2 tablespoons almond butter
- 2 tablespoons ground flaxseed

Berry Protein Pack (makes 2 packs):

- 2 cups mixed frozen berries
- 2 tablespoons chia seeds
- 2 tablespoons vanilla protein powder (optional)
- 1/4 cup rolled oats

Tropical Coconut Pack (makes 2 packs):

- 1 cup frozen pineapple
- 1 cup frozen mango
- 1/4 cup coconut flakes
- 2 tablespoons coconut butter

Chocolate Almond Pack (makes 2 packs):

- 2 frozen bananas, sliced
- 4 tablespoons almond butter
- 2 tablespoons unsweetened cocoa powder
- 2 tablespoons chia seeds

DIRECTIONS

1. Divide ingredients for each pack type between 2 freezer-safe bags or containers.
2. Label each pack with contents and date.
3. Freeze for up to 3 months.
4. To make smoothie: Add contents of one pack to blender with 1-1.5 cups liquid of choice (almond milk, coconut milk, or water).
5. Blend until smooth, adding more liquid as needed for desired consistency.
6. Pour into glass and enjoy immediately.

Baked Oatmeal Squares

Cut into portable squares, this baked oatmeal provides the comfort of a warm breakfast with the convenience of grab-and-go portability.

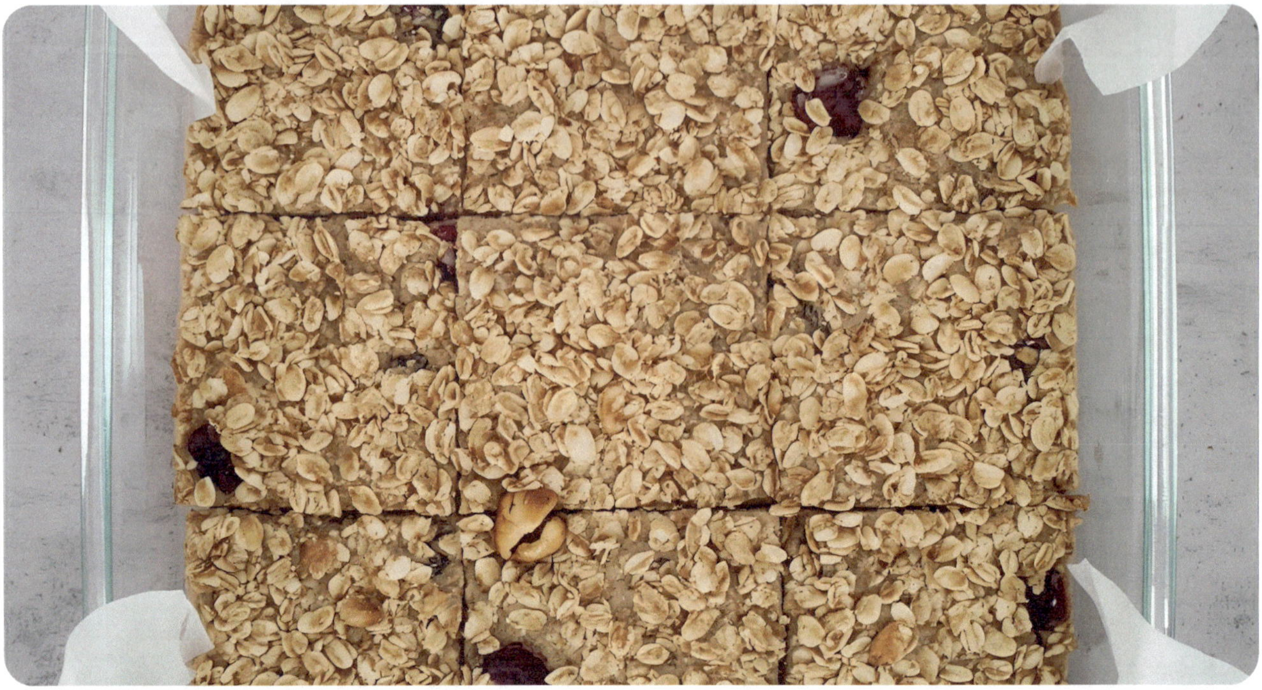

DIRECTIONS

1. Preheat oven to 350°F (175°C). Spray an 8x8-inch baking dish with cooking spray.
2. In a large bowl, combine oats, walnuts, baking powder, cinnamon, salt, and nutmeg.
3. In another bowl, whisk together almond milk, maple syrup, eggs, melted coconut oil, and vanilla.
4. Pour wet ingredients over dry ingredients and stir until combined.
5. Fold in berries gently.
6. Pour mixture into prepared baking dish and spread evenly.
7. Bake for 35-40 minutes until top is golden and center is set.
8. Cool completely before cutting into 9 squares.

9 | 15 minutes | 35 minutes

NUTRITION

Per serving: 215 calories, 7g protein, 32g carbohydrates, 8g fat, 5g fiber

STORAGE

Refrigerate for up to 5 days or freeze individual squares for up to 3 months. Reheat in microwave for 30-60 seconds.

INGREDIENTS

- 3 cups rolled oats (certified gluten-free)
- 1/3 cup chopped walnuts
- 1 teaspoon baking powder
- 1 teaspoon cinnamon
- 1/2 teaspoon salt
- 1/4 teaspoon nutmeg
- 1 cup unsweetened almond milk
- 1/3 cup sugar free maple syrup
- 2 large eggs
- 3 tablespoons melted coconut oil
- 2 teaspoons vanilla extract
- 1 1/2 cups mixed berries (fresh or frozen)
- Cooking spray

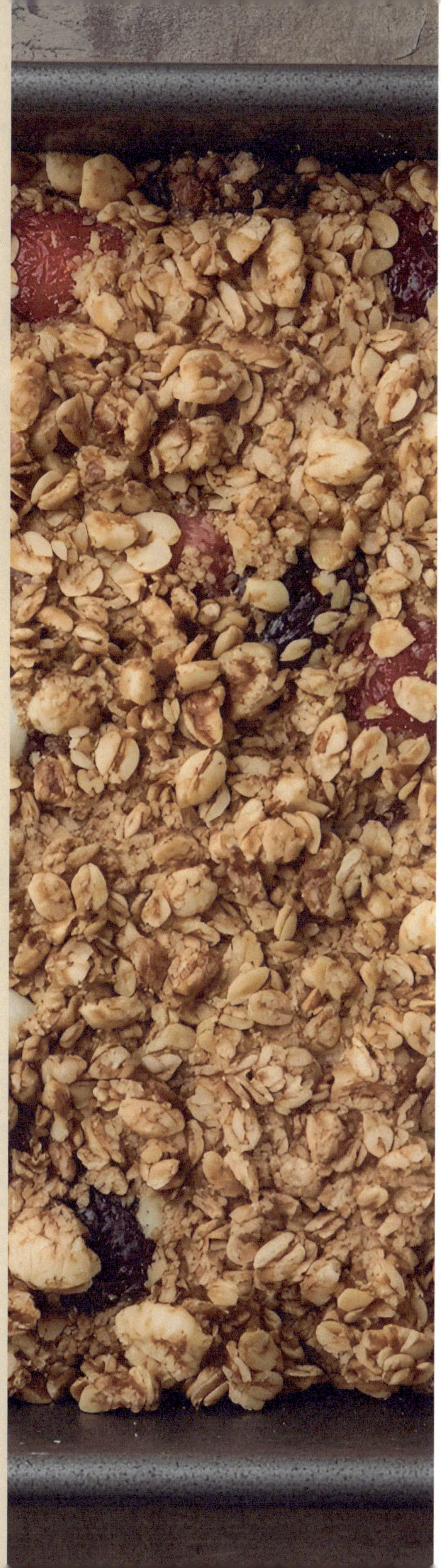

Tips For Success

Batch Prep on Weekends: Dedicate 2-3 hours on Sunday to prepare multiple breakfast options for the week. Having variety prevents boredom and ensures you'll stick to your healthy eating goals.

Proper Storage is Key: Invest in quality glass containers and freezer bags. Label everything with contents and date to maintain a well-organized system.

Customize for Your Household: Double recipes if you have a large family, or halve them if you're cooking for one or two people.

Rotation Strategy: Prepare 2-3 different make-ahead options each week to provide variety and prevent breakfast fatigue.

Emergency Backup: Always keep 2-3 frozen breakfast options available for weeks when life gets particularly hectic.

Test and Adjust: Try each recipe once on a weekend when you have time to adjust flavors or textures before committing to a full week's menu.

Remember, the goal is to make your mornings easier, not to create additional stress. Start with one or two make-ahead options and gradually build your repertoire as these become routine parts of your meal prep.

CHAPTER 05

Nourishing Soups and Stews

Soups and stews offer unparalleled comfort while providing some of the most blood sugar-friendly meals possible. The combination of protein, fiber-rich vegetables, and healthy fats in liquid form creates natural portion control while maximizing satiety and nutrient absorption. These recipes prove that gluten-free soups need never rely on flour-based thickeners when vegetables, beans, and natural reduction techniques can create body and richness. From light, broth-based soups perfect for warm weather to hearty stews that satisfy on the coldest days, these recipes provide nourishment that feels like a warm embrace while supporting your health goals.

List of Recipes

1. White Bean and Kale Soup
2. Beef and Mushroom Stew
3. Hearty Fish Chowder
4. Turkish Red Lentil Soup
5. Coconut Curry Vegetable Soup
6. Classic Chicken and Vegetable Soup
7. Roasted Tomato Basil Soup
8. Chilled Cucumber Avocado Soup

White Bean and Kale Soup

Servings	Prep time	Cook time
6	15 minutes	25 minutes

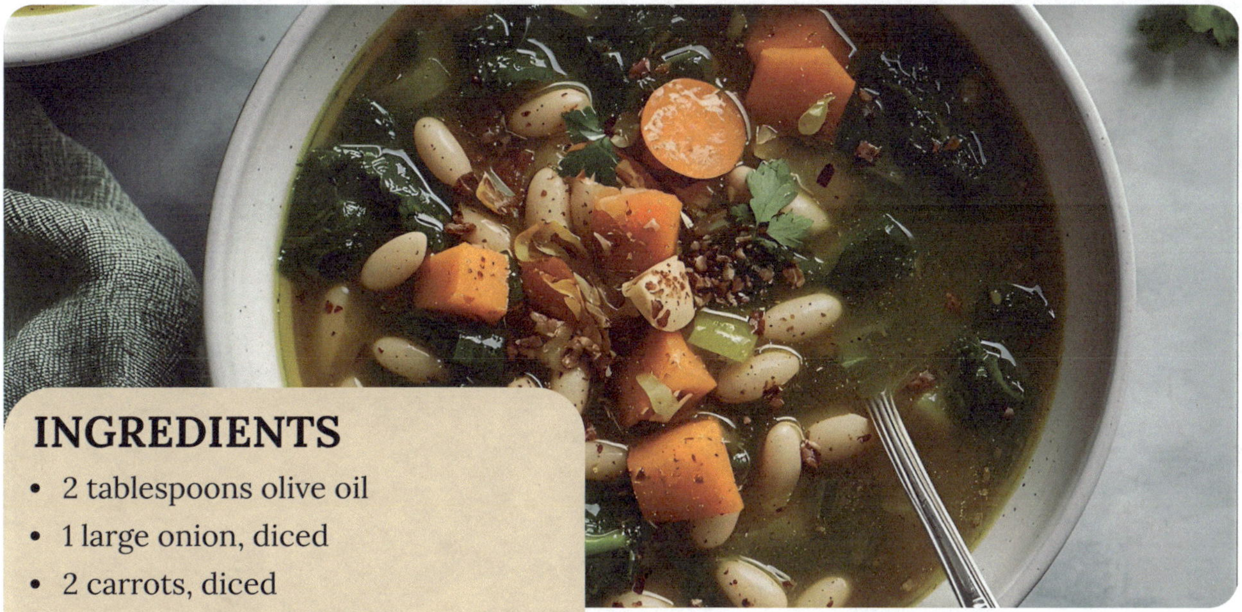

INGREDIENTS

- 2 tablespoons olive oil
- 1 large onion, diced
- 2 carrots, diced
- 2 celery stalks, diced
- 4 cloves garlic, minced
- 1 teaspoon dried oregano
- 1/4 teaspoon red pepper flakes
- 6 cups low-sodium vegetable broth
- 2 cans (15 oz each) white beans, drained and rinsed
- 4 cups kale, stems removed and leaves chopped
- 2 tablespoons lemon juice
- 1/4 cup fresh parsley, chopped
- Salt and black pepper to taste
- Extra virgin olive oil for drizzling

NUTRITION

Per serving: 195 calories, 11g protein, 30g carbohydrates, 5g fat, 9g fiber

STORAGE

Refrigerate for up to 5 days or freeze for up to 3 months.

A nutritious, fiber-rich soup that combines protein-packed beans with nutrient-dense kale in a flavorful, satisfying broth.

DIRECTIONS

1. Heat olive oil in large pot over medium heat. Add onion, carrots, and celery. Cook 8 minutes until vegetables soften.
2. Add garlic, oregano, and red pepper flakes. Cook 1 minute until fragrant.
3. Add broth and beans. Bring to boil, then reduce heat and simmer 10 minutes.
4. Using back of spoon, mash some beans against side of pot to thicken soup slightly.
5. Add kale and simmer 5 minutes until wilted and tender.
6. Stir in lemon juice and parsley. Season with salt and pepper.
7. Serve hot, drizzled with extra virgin olive oil.

Beef & Mushroom Stew

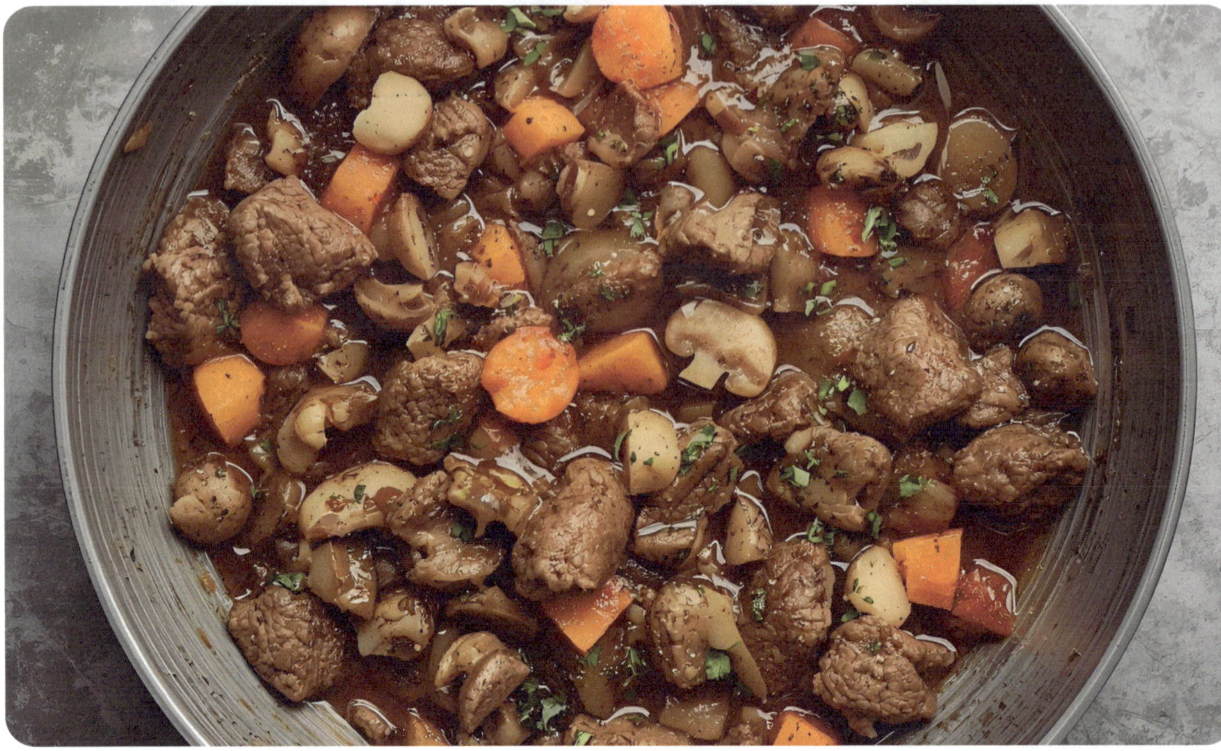

A rich, hearty stew that develops deep, complex flavors through slow braising, proving that gluten-free cooking can be every bit as satisfying as traditional versions.

8	25 minutes	2 hour

INGREDIENTS

- 3 lbs beef chuck roast, cut into 2-inch cubes
- 3 tablespoons olive oil
- 1 large onion, diced
- 1 lb mixed mushrooms (cremini, shiitake, oyster), sliced
- 4 cloves garlic, minced
- 2 tablespoons tomato paste
- 1 cup red wine (optional, or additional broth)
- 4 cups beef broth
- 2 bay leaves
- 2 sprigs fresh thyme
- 3 large carrots, cut into 2-inch pieces
- 1 lb small potatoes, halved
- 2 tablespoons fresh parsley, chopped
- Salt and black pepper to taste

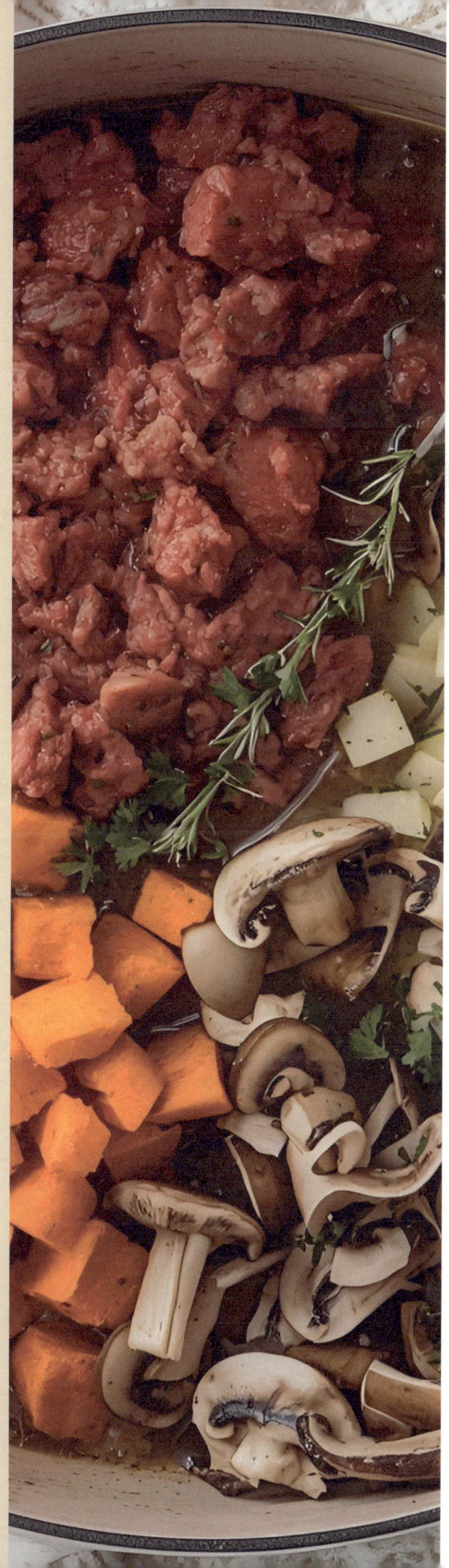

DIRECTION

1. Season beef cubes generously with salt and pepper.
2. Heat 2 tablespoons oil in large Dutch oven over medium-high heat. Brown beef in batches, about 8 minutes total. Remove and set aside.
3. Add remaining oil to pot. Add onion and cook 5 minutes until softened.
4. Add mushrooms and cook 8 minutes until liquid evaporates and mushrooms are golden.
5. Add garlic and tomato paste, cooking 2 minutes until fragrant.
6. Add wine (if using) and scrape up browned bits. Cook 3 minutes.
7. Return beef to pot and add broth, bay leaves, and thyme. Bring to boil.
8. Reduce heat to low, cover, and simmer 1 hour.
9. Add carrots and potatoes. Continue simmering 45 minutes until beef is tender.
10. Remove bay leaves and thyme stems. Stir in parsley and adjust seasoning. Serve hot.

NUTRITION

Per serving: 385 calories, 32g protein, 18g carbohydrates, 19g fat, 3g fiber

STORAGE

Refrigerate for up to 4 days or freeze for up to 4 months.

Hearty Fish Chowder

A rich, satisfying chowder that achieves creaminess through pureed vegetables rather than flour or heavy cream, keeping it both gluten-free and lighter.

INGREDIENTS

- 2 tablespoons olive oil
- 4 slices bacon, chopped (optional)
- 1 large onion, diced
- 2 celery stalks, diced
- 2 medium potatoes, peeled and cubed
- 3 cloves garlic, minced
- 1 bay leaf
- 1 teaspoon dried thyme
- 4 cups fish stock or low-sodium chicken broth
- 1 cup unsweetened almond milk
- 1 1/2 lbs firm white fish (cod, halibut, or haddock), cut into chunks
- 1 cup corn kernels (fresh or frozen)
- 2 tablespoons fresh parsley, chopped
- 2 tablespoons lemon juice
- Salt and black pepper to taste

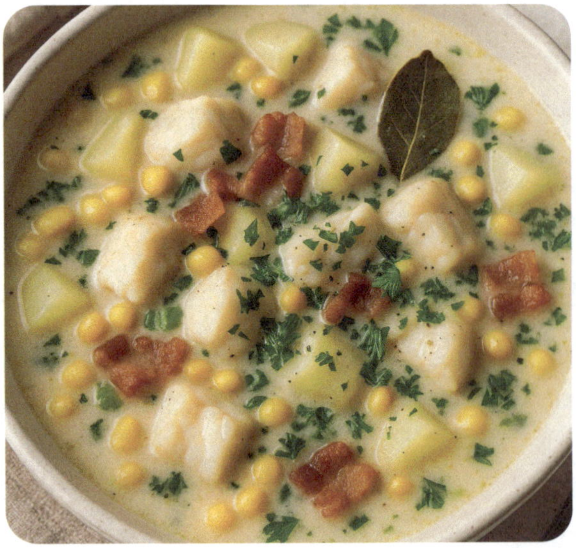

6 | 20 minutes | 35 minutes

DIRECTIONS

1. Heat olive oil in large pot over medium heat. Add bacon (if using) and cook until crispy. Remove with slotted spoon.
2. Add onion and celery to pot and cook 6 minutes until softened.
3. Add half the potatoes, garlic, bay leaf, and thyme. Cook 2 minutes.
4. Add broth and bring to boil. Reduce heat and simmer 15 minutes until potatoes are very tender.
5. Remove bay leaf. Using immersion blender, partially puree soup, leaving some chunks for texture.
6. Add remaining potatoes and almond milk. Simmer 10 minutes until potatoes are tender.
7. Gently add fish and corn. Simmer 5-7 minutes until fish is cooked through.
8. Stir in parsley, lemon juice, and reserved bacon (if using). Season with salt and pepper.
9. Serve hot.

NUTRITION

Per serving: 225 calories, 26g protein, 18g carbohydrates, 6g fat, 2g fiber

STORAGE

Refrigerate for up to 2 days. Do not freeze as fish texture will suffer

Turkish Red Lentil Soup

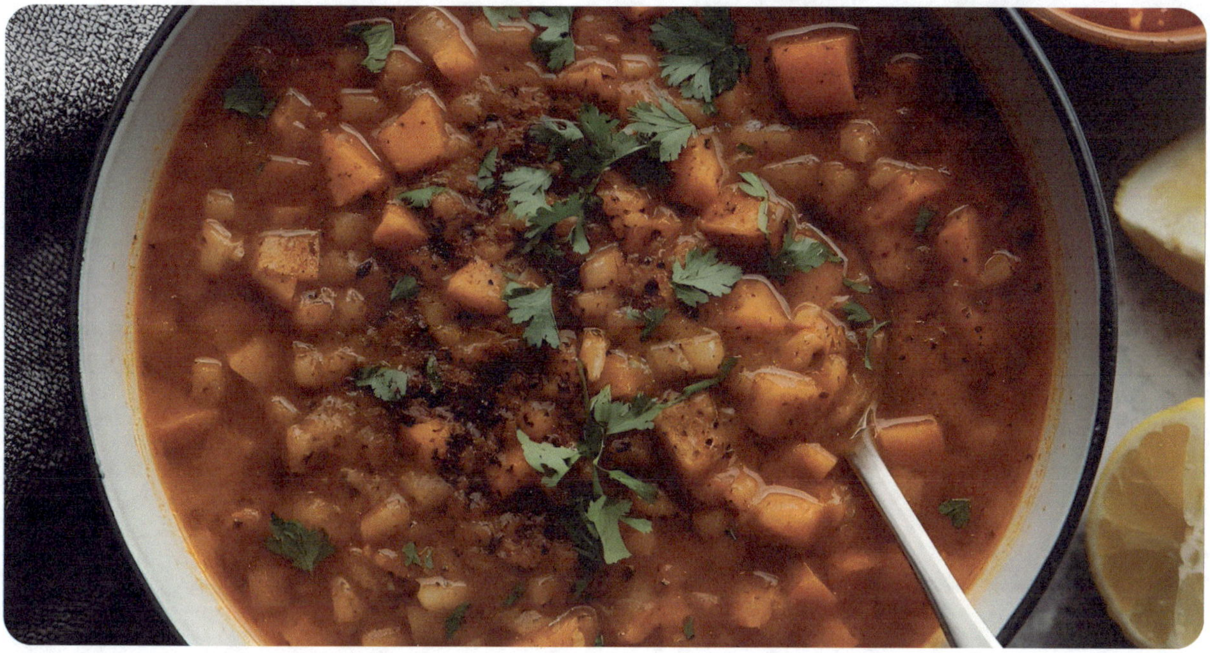

A protein-rich, warming soup with Middle Eastern flavors that becomes silky and satisfying as the lentils break down during cooking.

Servings	Prep time	Cook time
6	15 minutes	30 minutes

INGREDIENTS

- 2 tablespoons olive oil
- 1 large onion, diced
- 2 carrots, diced
- 3 cloves garlic, minced
- 1 tablespoon tomato paste
- 1 teaspoon ground cumin
- 1 teaspoon paprika
- 1/2 teaspoon turmeric
- 1/4 teaspoon cayenne pepper
- 1 1/2 cups red lentils, rinsed
- 6 cups low-sodium vegetable broth
- 1 bay leaf
- 2 tablespoons lemon juice
- Salt and black pepper to taste
- Fresh cilantro for garnish
- Lemon wedges for serving

DIRECTIONS

1. Heat olive oil in large pot over medium heat. Add onion and carrots, cooking 8 minutes until softened.
2. Add garlic, tomato paste, cumin, paprika, turmeric, and cayenne. Cook 2 minutes until fragrant.
3. Add lentils, broth, and bay leaf. Bring to boil.
4. Reduce heat and simmer 20-25 minutes until lentils are very soft and soup is thickened.
5. Remove bay leaf. Using immersion blender, partially blend soup, leaving some texture.
6. Stir in lemon juice and season with salt and pepper.
7. Garnish with cilantro and serve with lemon wedges.

NUTRITION

Per serving: 215 calories, 13g protein, 35g carbohydrates, 4g fat, 7g fiber

STORAGE

Refrigerate for up to 5 days or freeze for up to 3 months. Add water when reheating if needed.

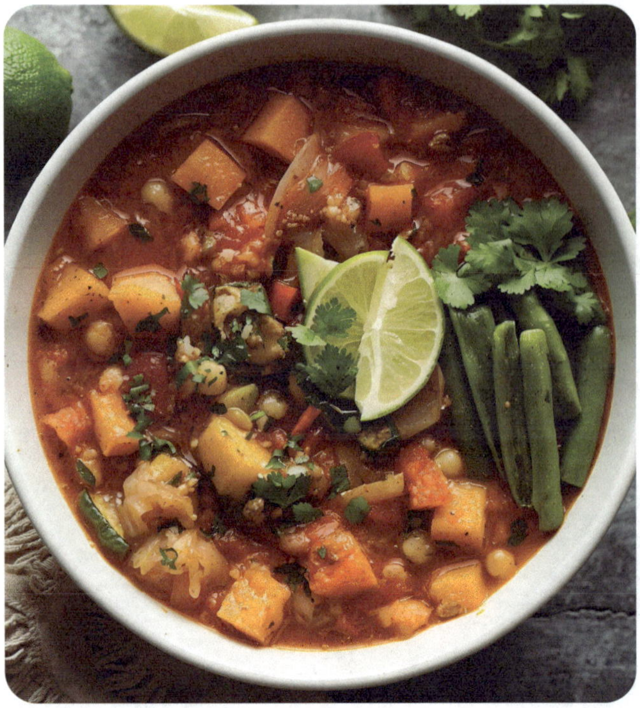

Coconut Curry Vegetable Soup

A vibrant, warming soup that combines coconut milk's richness with aromatic spices and fresh vegetables for a satisfying plant-based meal.

Servings	Prep time	Cook time
5	20 minutes	25 minutes

NUTRITION

Per serving: 245 calories, 8g protein, 24g carbohydrates, 14g fat, 7g fiber

STORAGE

Refrigerate for up to 4 days. Do not freeze due to coconut milk separation.

INGREDIENTS

- 2 tablespoons coconut oil
- 1 large onion, diced
- 1 red bell pepper, diced
- 3 cloves garlic, minced
- 1 tablespoon fresh ginger, minced
- 2 tablespoons red curry paste
- 1 can (14 oz) coconut milk
- 3 cups low-sodium vegetable broth
- 1 sweet potato, peeled and cubed
- 1 zucchini, diced
- 1 cup green beans, trimmed and cut into 1-inch pieces
- 1 can (15 oz) chickpeas, drained and rinsed
- 2 tablespoons lime juice
- 1/4 cup fresh cilantro, chopped
- Salt to taste
- Lime wedges for serving

DIRECTIONS

1. Heat coconut oil in large pot over medium heat. Add onion and bell pepper, cooking 6 minutes until softened.
2. Add garlic, ginger, and curry paste. Cook 2 minutes until fragrant.
3. Stir in coconut milk and broth, scraping up any browned bits.
4. Add sweet potato and bring to boil. Reduce heat and simmer 10 minutes.
5. Add zucchini, green beans, and chickpeas. Simmer 10 minutes more until vegetables are tender.
6. Stir in lime juice and cilantro. Season with salt.
7. Serve hot with lime wedges.

Classic Chicken & Vegetable Soup

INGREDIENTS

- 2 tablespoons olive oil
- 1 large onion, diced
- 3 carrots, sliced into rounds
- 3 celery stalks, diced
- 3 cloves garlic, minced
- 8 cups low-sodium chicken broth
- 1 lb boneless, skinless chicken thighs, cut into bite-sized pieces
- 2 bay leaves
- 1 teaspoon dried thyme
- 1/2 teaspoon dried oregano
- 1 cup green beans, trimmed and cut into 1-inch pieces
- 1/2 cup fresh parsley, chopped
- Salt and black pepper to taste
- 2 tablespoons lemon juice

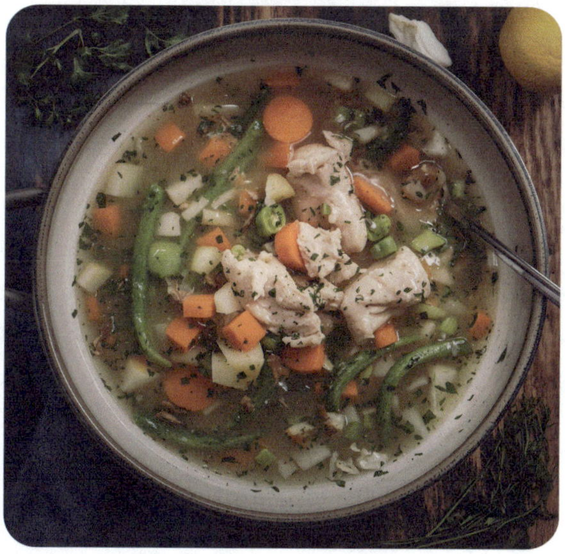

A timeless comfort soup that proves simple ingredients can create deeply satisfying meals when treated with care and patience.

8 | 20 minutes | 45 minutes

DIRECTIONS

1. Heat olive oil in large pot over medium heat. Add onion, carrots, and celery. Cook 8-10 minutes until vegetables soften.
2. Add garlic and cook 1 minute until fragrant.
3. Add chicken broth, chicken pieces, bay leaves, thyme, and oregano. Bring to boil.
4. Reduce heat and simmer 20 minutes until chicken is cooked through.
5. Add green beans and simmer 10 minutes more until tender.
6. Remove bay leaves. Stir in parsley and lemon juice.
7. Season with salt and pepper to taste.
8. Serve hot.

NUTRITION

Per serving: 165 calories, 18g protein, 8g carbohydrates, 6g fat, 2g fiber

STORAGE

Refrigerate for up to 4 days or freeze for up to 3 months.

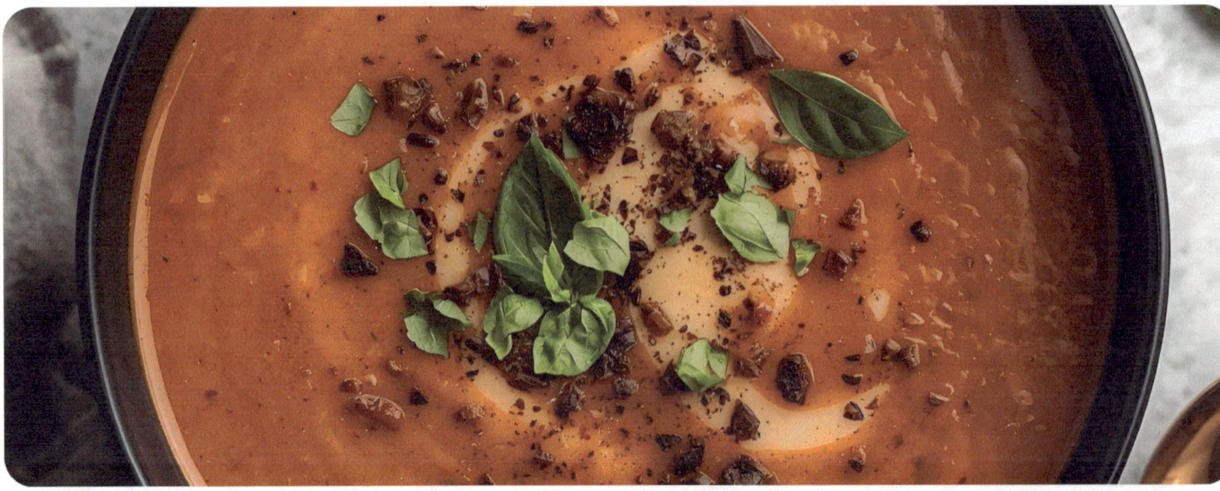

Roasted Tomato Basil Soup

6 | 15 minutes | 45 minutes

INGREDIENTS

- 3 lbs ripe tomatoes, halved
- 1 large onion, quartered
- 4 cloves garlic, unpeeled
- 3 tablespoons olive oil
- 3 cups low-sodium vegetable broth
- 1/4 cup fresh basil leaves, plus more for garnish
- 1 tablespoon balsamic vinegar
- 1 teaspoon salt
- 1/2 teaspoon black pepper
- 1/4 teaspoon red pepper flakes (optional)

Roasting the tomatoes intensifies their natural sweetness and creates a rich, velvety soup without any cream or flour.

DIRECTIONS

1. Preheat oven to 425°F (220°C).
2. Place tomatoes cut-side down on large baking sheet with onion and garlic. Drizzle with 2 tablespoons olive oil.
3. Roast 35-40 minutes until tomatoes are caramelized and onions are tender.
4. Cool slightly, then peel garlic cloves.
5. Transfer roasted vegetables to blender or food processor. Add 1 cup broth and blend until smooth.
6. Pour into large pot and add remaining broth, basil, balsamic vinegar, salt, pepper, and red pepper flakes.
7. Simmer 10 minutes to blend flavors.
8. Drizzle with remaining olive oil and garnish with fresh basil before serving.

NUTRITION

Per serving: 95 calories, 3g protein, 12g carbohydrates, 5g fat, 3g fiber

STORAGE

Refrigerate for up to 5 days or freeze for up to 4 months.

Chilled Cucumber Avocado Soup

A refreshing cold soup perfect for warm weather, combining cooling cucumber with creamy avocado and bright herbs.

Servings	Prep time	Cook time
4	15 minutes plus 2 hours chilling	0 minutes

INGREDIENTS

- 3 large English cucumbers, peeled and roughly chopped
- 2 ripe avocados, pitted and peeled
- 1 cup unsweetened coconut milk (canned)
- 1/4 cup fresh lime juice
- 1/4 cup fresh mint leaves
- 2 tablespoons fresh dill
- 1 clove garlic, minced
- 1 teaspoon salt
- 1/4 teaspoon white pepper
- 1/2 cup cold water as needed
- Extra cucumber, diced, for garnish
- Fresh herbs for garnish
- Lime wedges for serving

DIRECTIONS

1. In a blender or food processor, combine cucumbers, avocados, coconut milk, lime juice, mint, dill, garlic, salt, and white pepper.
2. Blend until completely smooth, adding cold water as needed to reach desired consistency.
3. Taste and adjust seasoning with additional lime juice, salt, or herbs as needed.
4. Refrigerate for at least 2 hours until well chilled.
5. Serve in chilled bowls, garnished with diced cucumber and fresh herbs.
6. Provide lime wedges for additional brightness.

NUTRITION

Per serving: 165 calories, 4g protein, 12g carbohydrates, 13g fat, 7g fiber

STORAGE

Best consumed within 24 hours. Stir before serving as separation may occur

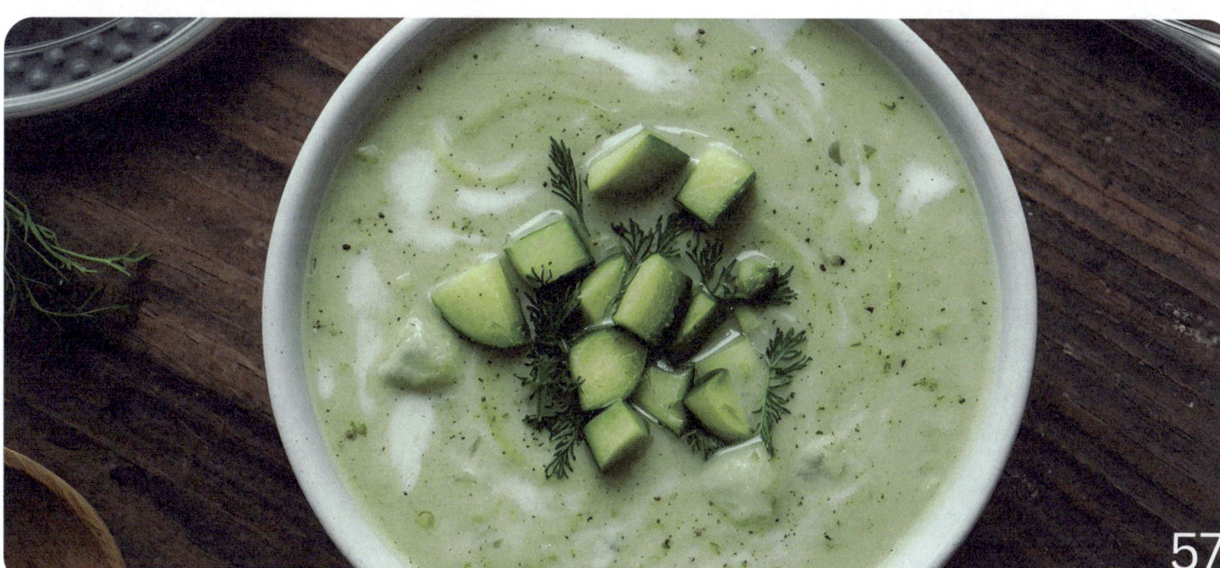

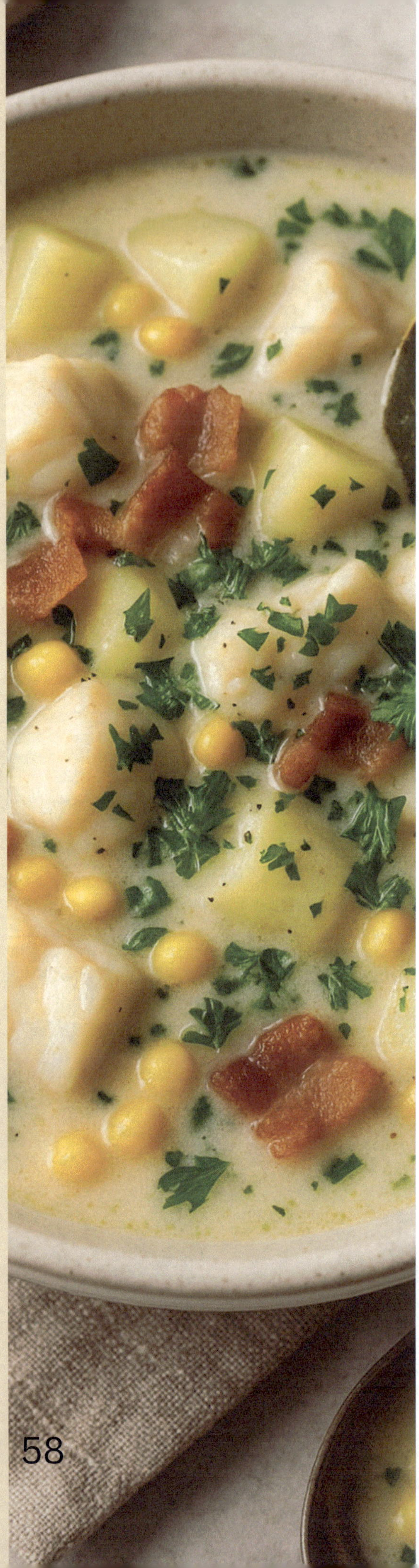

TIPS FOR PERFECT SOUPS AND STEW

Building Flavor Layers: Start with aromatic vegetables (onions, carrots, celery) cooked in fat, add garlic and spices, then liquid. Each step builds complexity that can't be achieved by simply combining ingredients.

Natural Thickening: Use pureed beans, vegetables, or potatoes instead of flour-based roux. Partially blending soups creates body while maintaining texture interest.

Seasoning Throughout: Season at multiple stages of cooking rather than just at the end. Taste and adjust frequently, especially after adding liquid.

Make-Ahead Advantages: Most soups and stews improve overnight as flavors meld. Cool completely before refrigerating and skim any fat that solidifies on top before reheating.

Freezing Guidelines: Soups with dairy, coconut milk, or fish don't freeze well. Bean, vegetable, and meat-based soups freeze beautifully for up to 3 months.

Portion Control: Soup naturally provides portion control and satiety. Start meals with broth-based soups to help manage hunger and blood sugar.

Fresh Finish: Add fresh herbs, citrus juice, or a drizzle of good olive oil just before serving to brighten flavors and add visual appeal.

Storage Solutions: Invest in quality freezer containers or bags. Freeze in family-sized or individual portions for maximum convenience.

Remember that soup-making is forgiving and adaptable. Use these recipes as starting points and adjust vegetables, proteins, and seasonings based on your preferences and what's available seasonally.

CHAPTER 06

Vibrant Salads and Grain Bowls

Gone are the days when salads meant iceberg lettuce with a few sad vegetables on the side. These recipes transform salads and bowls into substantial, satisfying meals that celebrate seasonal produce, interesting textures, and bold flavor combinations. Each bowl is designed to provide complete nutrition – protein, healthy fats, complex carbohydrates, and plenty of fiber – while keeping blood sugar stable and energy sustained. The homemade dressings featured throughout this chapter eliminate he hidden sugars and preservatives found in most commercial versions, giving you complete control over flavor and nutrition while often tasting far superior to anything you can buy.

List of Recipes

1. Roasted Beet and Goat Cheese Salad
2. Asian Inspired Cabbage Slaw
3. Rice Salad with Cranberries and Pecans
4. Mediterranean Chickpea Power Salad
5. Mexican Street Corn Salad Bowl
6. Thai-Style Beef Salad
7. Spiralized Beet and Citrus Salad

Roasted Beet and Goat Cheese Salad

4 | 15 minutes | 45 minutes

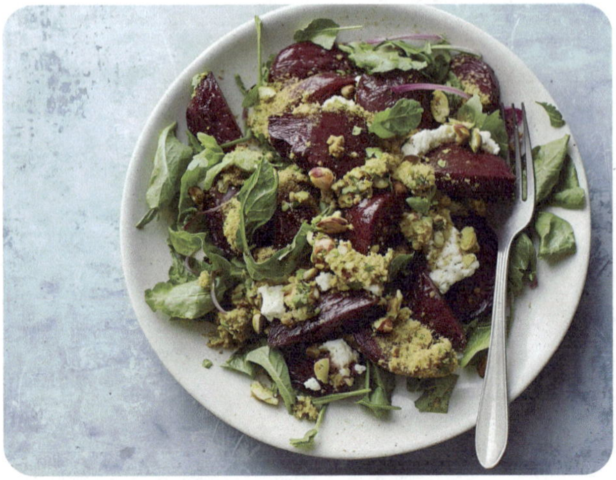

This elegant salad combines classic beet and goat cheese pairing with unexpected citrus brightness and the subtle licorice notes of tarragon.

INGREDIENTS

For the salad:

- 4 medium beets, trimmed and scrubbed
- 4 cups mixed greens (arugula, spinach, spring mix)
- 4 oz goat cheese, crumbled
- 1/3 cup pistachios, shelled and roughly chopped
- 2 tablespoons fresh tarragon, chopped

For orange-tarragon vinaigrette:

- 3 tablespoons olive oil
- 2 tablespoons fresh orange juice
- 1 tablespoon white wine vinegar
- 1 teaspoon orange zest
- 1 teaspoon fresh tarragon, minced
- 1/2 teaspoon Dijon mustard
- 1/4 teaspoon salt
- 1/8 teaspoon black pepper

DIRECTIONS

1. Preheat oven to 400°F (200°C). Wrap each beet individually in foil and roast 45-60 minutes until tender when pierced with knife.
2. Cool beets, then peel and slice into wedges.
3. Make vinaigrette: Whisk together olive oil, orange juice, white wine vinegar, orange zest, tarragon, Dijon mustard, salt, and pepper.
4. Arrange mixed greens on serving plates.
5. Top with roasted beet wedges and crumbled goat cheese.
6. Drizzle with vinaigrette and sprinkle with pistachios and fresh tarragon.
7. Serve immediately.

NUTRITION

Per serving: 215 calories, 9g protein, 14g carbohydrates, 15g fat, 4g fiber

STORAGE

Roasted beets can be prepared up to 3 days ahead. Assemble salad just before serving.

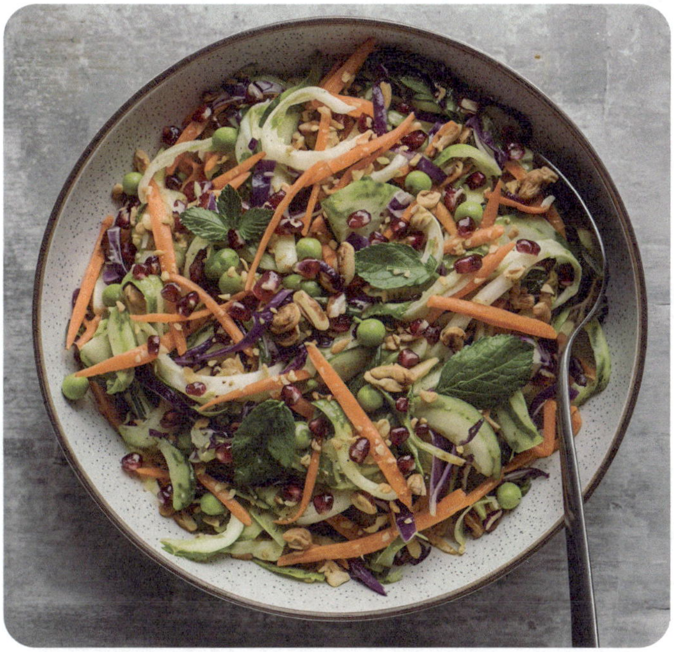

Asian Inspired Cabbage Slaw with Peanut Dressing

This crunchy, refreshing slaw gets an unexpected twist from juicy pomegranate seeds and cooling mint that elevate it beyond typical Asian salads.

Servings	Prep time	Cook time
6	20 minutes	0 minutes

NUTRITION

Per serving: 165 calories, 8g protein, 15g carbohydrates, 9g fat, 5g fiber

STORAGE

Slaw keeps for up to 2 days in refrigerator. Add pomegranate seeds and herbs just before serving.

INGREDIENTS

For the slaw:

- 4 cups napa cabbage, thinly sliced
- 2 cups red cabbage, thinly sliced
- 2 large carrots, julienned
- 1 red bell pepper, thinly sliced
- 1 cup edamame, shelled and cooked
- 1/2 cup pomegranate seeds
- 1/4 cup fresh mint leaves, chopped
- 1/4 cup fresh cilantro, chopped
- 1/3 cup roasted peanuts, roughly chopped

For peanut dressing:

- 3 tablespoons natural peanut butter
- 2 tablespoons rice vinegar
- 1 tablespoon sesame oil
- 1 tablespoon low-sodium soy sauce (gluten-free)
- 1 tablespoon lime juice
- 1 teaspoon fresh ginger, grated
- 1 clove garlic, minced
- 1 teaspoon honey
- 2-3 tablespoons warm water to thin

DIRECTIONS

1. Make Dressing: In small bowl, whisk together peanut butter, rice vinegar, sesame oil, soy sauce, lime juice, ginger, garlic, and honey. Add warm water gradually until desired consistency.
2. Make Salad: In large bowl, combine both cabbages, carrots, bell pepper, and edamame.
3. Add dressing and toss until vegetables are well coated.
4. Let sit 10 minutes for flavors to meld.
5. Just before serving, add pomegranate seeds, mint, and cilantro. Toss gently.
6. Top with roasted peanuts and serve immediately.

Warm Wild Rice Salad with Cranberries and Pecans

Servings	Prep time	Cook time
6	15 minutes	45 minutes

A timeless comfort salad that proves simple ingredients can create deeply satisfying meals when treated with care and patience.

INGREDIENTS

For the salad:

- 1 1/2 cups wild rice
- 4 cups low-sodium chicken or vegetable broth
- 1/2 cup dried cranberries (no sugar added)
- 1/2 cup pecans, toasted and roughly chopped
- 2 celery stalks, finely diced
- 1/4 cup fresh parsley, chopped
- 2 green onions, sliced

For maple-Dijon dressing:

- 3 tablespoons olive oil
- 2 tablespoons apple cider vinegar
- 1 tablespoon sugar free maple syrup
- 1 tablespoon Dijon mustard
- 1/2 teaspoon salt
- 1/4 teaspoon black pepper
- 1/4 teaspoon dried thyme

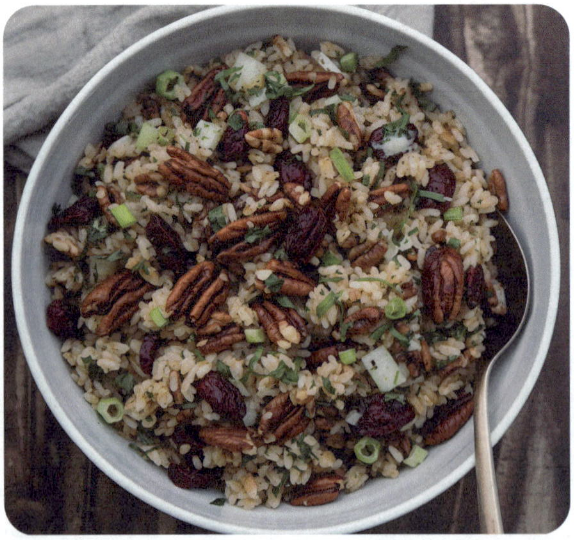

DIRECTIONS

1. Cook wild rice in broth according to package directions (about 45 minutes). Drain any excess liquid and let cool slightly.
2. Make dressing: Whisk together olive oil, apple cider vinegar, maple syrup, Dijon mustard, salt, pepper, and thyme.
3. In large bowl, combine warm wild rice with cranberries (the warmth will plump them slightly).
4. Add celery, parsley, and green onions.
5. Pour dressing over salad and toss to combine.
6. Top with toasted pecans just before serving.
7. Serve warm or at room temperature.

NUTRITION

Per serving: 285 calories, 8g protein, 42g carbohydrates, 11g fat, 4g fiber

STORAGE

Keeps for up to 4 days in refrigerator. Best served at room temperature.

Mediterranean Chickpea Power Salad

6	20 minutes	0 minutes

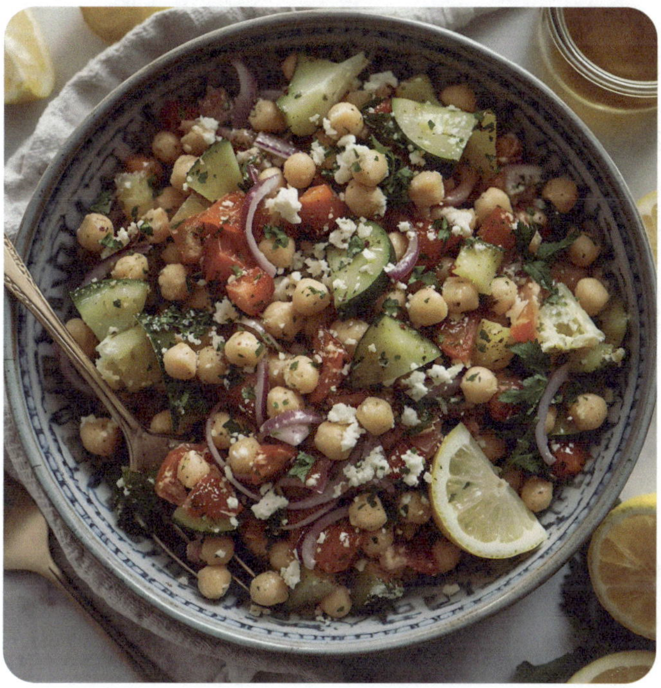

A protein-packed salad that gets better as it sits, making it perfect for meal prep and potluck gatherings.

DIRECTIONS

1. Make dressing: Whisk together olive oil, lemon juice, red wine vinegar, oregano, garlic, salt, and pepper.
2. In large bowl, combine chickpeas, cucumber, tomatoes, bell pepper, and red onion.
3. Add dressing and toss to combine.
4. Let marinate 15 minutes at room temperature.
5. Add parsley and mint, toss gently.
6. Top with feta cheese before serving.
7. Serve at room temperature or chilled.

INGREDIENTS

For the salad:

- 2 cans (15 oz each) chickpeas, drained and rinsed
- 1 English cucumber, diced
- 1 cup cherry tomatoes, halved
- 1/2 red bell pepper, diced
- 1/2 cup red onion, finely diced
- 1/2 cup fresh parsley, chopped
- 1/4 cup fresh mint, chopped
- 1/3 cup feta cheese, crumbled

For lemon-oregano dressing:

- 1/4 cup extra virgin olive oil
- 3 tablespoons fresh lemon juice
- 1 tablespoon red wine vinegar
- 2 teaspoons dried oregano
- 1 clove garlic, minced
- 1/2 teaspoon salt
- 1/4 teaspoon black pepper

NUTRITION

Per serving: 215 calories, 9g protein, 24g carbohydrates, 10g fat, 7g fiber

STORAGE

Keeps for up to 4 days in refrigerator. Add herbs and feta just before serving.

Mexican Street Corn Salad Bowl

All the flavors of Mexican street corn transformed into a satisfying grain bowl with brown rice and black beans for complete protein.

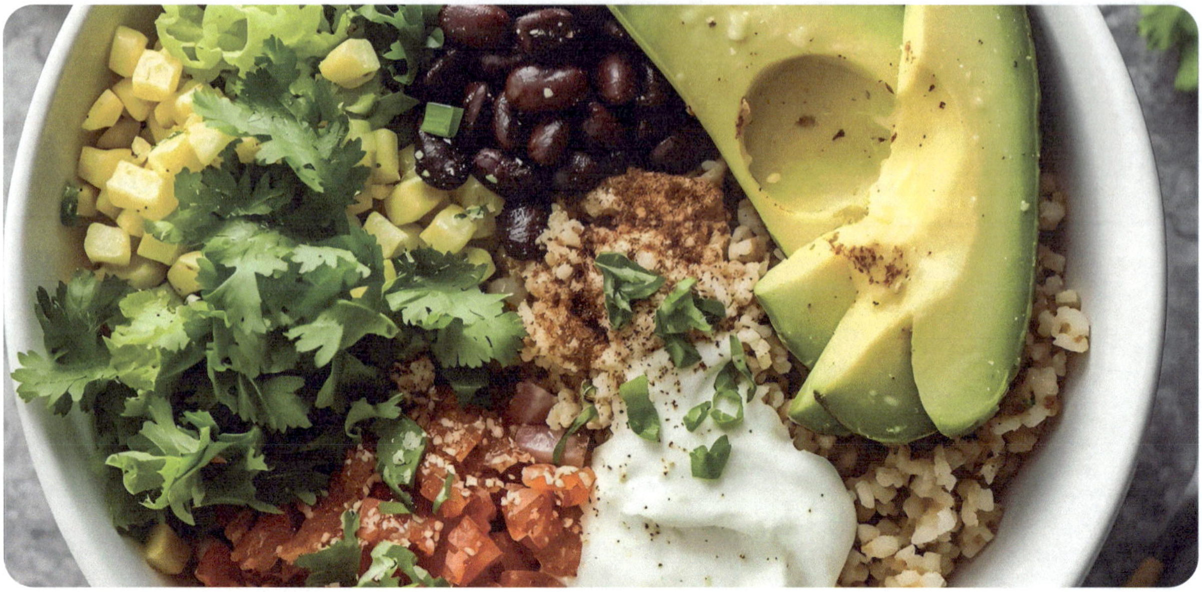

INGREDIENTS

For the bowl:

- 2 cups cooked brown rice, cooled
- 4 ears corn, kernels removed (about 3 cups)
- 1 can (15 oz) black beans, drained and rinsed
- 2 cups romaine lettuce, chopped
- 1 avocado, diced
- 1/4 cup red onion, finely diced
- 1/4 cup fresh cilantro, chopped
- 1/4 cup cotija cheese, crumbled

For lime-chili dressing:

- 1/4 cup plain Greek yogurt
- 2 tablespoons lime juice
- 1 tablespoon olive oil
- 1 clove garlic, minced
- 1/2 teaspoon chili powder
- 1/4 teaspoon ground cumin
- 1/4 teaspoon smoked paprika
- 1/4 teaspoon salt
- 1/8 teaspoon cayenne pepper

Servings	Prep time	Cook time
4	20 minutes	10 minutes

DIRECTIONS

1. Heat large skillet over medium-high heat. Add corn kernels and cook 6-8 minutes until slightly charred, stirring occasionally.
2. Make dressing: Whisk together Greek yogurt, lime juice, olive oil, garlic, chili powder, cumin, smoked paprika, salt, and cayenne.
3. In large bowl, combine brown rice, charred corn, and black beans.
4. Add half the dressing and toss to combine.
5. Divide romaine among 4 bowls. Top with rice mixture.
6. Add avocado, red onion, and cilantro.
7. Drizzle with remaining dressing and top with cotija cheese.

NUTRITION

Per serving: 385 calories, 16g protein, 65g carbohydrates, 9g fat, 12g fiber

STORAGE

Components can be prepared separately and stored for up to 2 days. Assemble just before serving.

Thai-Style Beef Salad

Servings	Prep time	Cook time
4	25 minutes	10 minutes

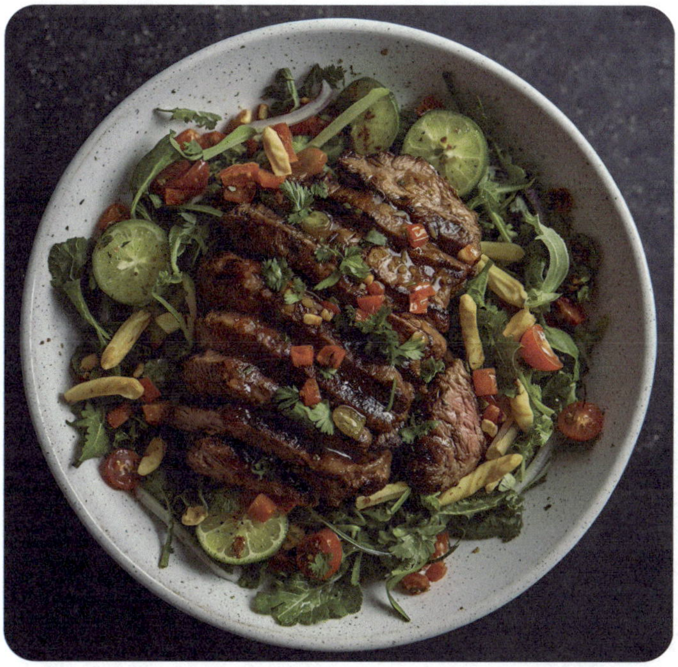

A bold, refreshing salad that combines perfectly seared beef with crisp vegetables and a tangy Thai-inspired dressing.

DIRECTIONS

1. Make dressing: Whisk together lime juice, fish sauce, rice vinegar, honey, garlic, and chili. Slowly whisk in olive oil.
2. Season steak with salt and pepper. Heat olive oil in large skillet over medium-high heat.
3. Cook steak 4-5 minutes per side for medium-rare. Rest 5 minutes, then slice thinly against the grain.
4. In large bowl, combine mixed greens, cucumber, tomatoes, red onion, mint, and cilantro.
5. Add half the dressing and toss gently.
6. Arrange salad on plates and top with sliced steak.
7. Drizzle with remaining dressing and sprinkle with peanuts.

INGREDIENTS

For the salad:

- 1 lb flank steak
- 6 cups mixed greens
- 1 cucumber, thinly sliced
- 1 cup cherry tomatoes, halved
- 1/2 red onion, thinly sliced
- 1/2 cup fresh mint leaves
- 1/2 cup fresh cilantro leaves
- 1/4 cup roasted peanuts, chopped

For Thai dressing:

- 3 tablespoons lime juice
- 2 tablespoons fish sauce
- 1 tablespoon rice vinegar
- 1 tablespoon honey
- 2 cloves garlic, minced
- 1 Thai chili, minced (or 1/4 teaspoon red pepper flakes)
- 2 tablespoons olive oil

For steak:

- 2 tablespoons olive oil
- Salt and black pepper

NUTRITION

Per serving: 295 calories, 26g protein, 12g carbohydrates, 16g fat, 3g fiber

STORAGE

Best served immediately.
Dressing can be made 1 day ahead.

Spiralized Beet & Citrus Salad

Servings	Prep time	Cook time
6	15 minutes	0 minutes

A vibrant salad of sweet beets, juicy citrus, crisp greens, and a refreshing mint finish.

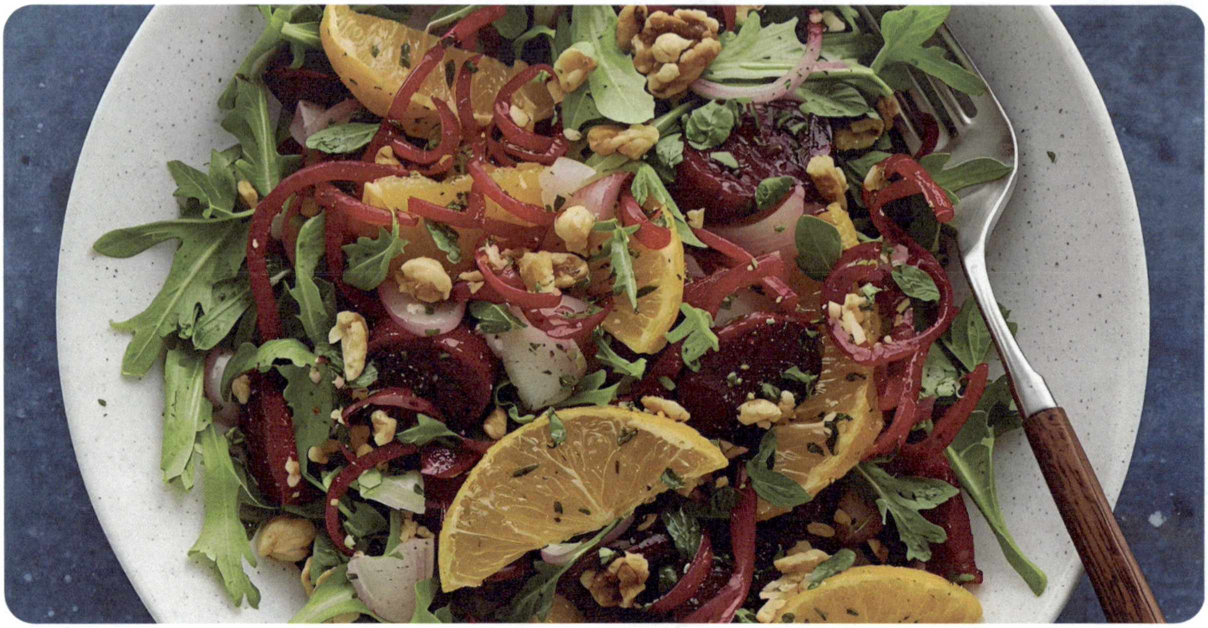

DIRECTIONS

1. In a large bowl, combine spiralized beets, orange segments, red onion, arugula, and walnuts.
2. In a small bowl, whisk olive oil, vinegar, honey, mustard, salt, and pepper.
3. Pour dressing over salad and toss gently to coat.
4. Sprinkle with fresh mint and serve immediately.

NUTRITION

Per serving: 125 calories, 3g protein, 13g carbohydrates, 8g fat, 3g fiber

STORAGE

Keeps for 1 day refrigerated; best served fresh for texture.

INGREDIENTS

- 3 medium beets, spiralized or julienned
- 2 oranges, peeled and segmented
- ½ small red onion, thinly sliced
- 3 cups baby arugula
- ¼ cup toasted walnuts, roughly chopped
- 2 tbsp olive oil
- 1 tbsp apple cider vinegar
- 1 tsp honey or erythritol
- ½ tsp Dijon mustard
- Salt and black pepper to taste
- 2 tbsp fresh mint, chopped

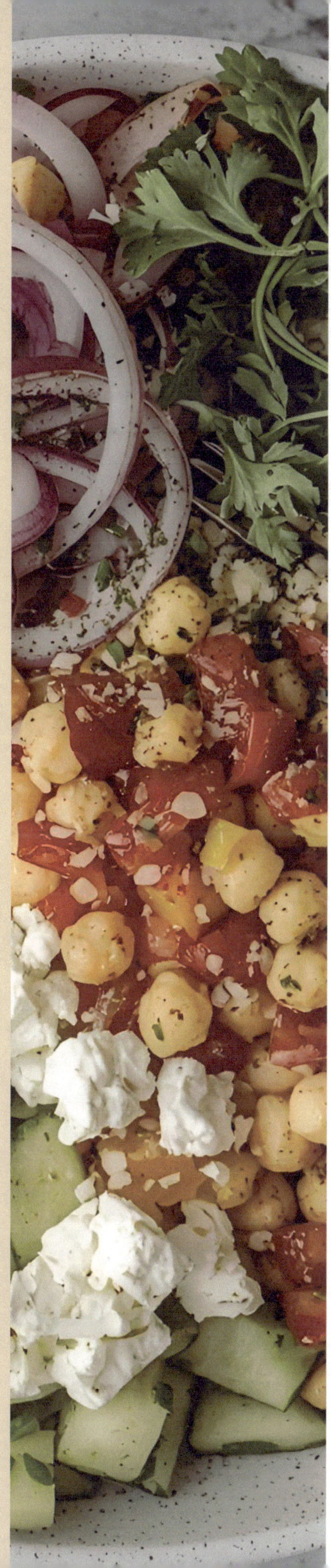

TIPS FOR PERFECT SALADS AND GRAIN BOWLS

Dressing Distribution: Always dress grains while they're still slightly warm to help absorption. For green salads, add dressing just before serving to prevent wilting.

Dressing Balance: Homemade dressings should balance acid (vinegar, citrus), fat (oil), and flavor enhancers (herbs, spices, mustard). Taste and adjust each element.

Texture Contrast: Combine different textures in each bowl - something crunchy (nuts, seeds, raw vegetables), something creamy (avocado, cheese, dressing), and something chewy (grains, dried fruit).

Temperature Play: Don't be afraid to combine warm and cool elements. Warm grains with cool vegetables, or room temperature proteins with chilled greens create interesting contrasts.

Make-Ahead Strategy: Prepare components separately and store in glass containers. Grains, proteins, and chopped vegetables keep well for 3-4 days. Add delicate elements like avocado and fresh herbs just before serving.

Seasoning Grains: Cook grains in broth instead of water when possible, and season the cooking liquid. This builds flavor from the foundation up.

Seasonal Adaptation: Use these recipes as templates and substitute seasonal vegetables and fruits to keep salads interesting year-round.

Storage Solutions: Glass meal prep containers work best for grain bowls as they don't absorb odors or stains. Keep dressings separate until serving to maintain optimal texture.

Protein Planning: Include at least one substantial protein source per bowl - beans, quinoa, nuts, seeds, eggs, or animal proteins. This ensures satiety and blood sugar stability.

CHAPTER 07

Comfort Food Classics Reimagined

List of Recipes

1. Polenta Rounds with Mushroom Ragout
2. Herb Crusted "Fried" Chicken
3. Cauliflower Mac and Cheese
4. Meatloaf with Mushroom Gravy
5. Chicken and Dumplings
6. Shepherd's Pie with Cauliflower Mash
7. Chicken Pot Pie with Almond Flour Crust
8. Tuna Noodle Casserole with Shitakes
9. Meatballs and Marinara
10. Chicken Parmesan with Zucchini
11. Black Bean and Quinoa Stuffed Peppers
12. Maple Roasted Pork Tenderloin
13. Herb Grilled Flank Steak with Wilted Greens
14. Asian Glazed Beef Skewers

Comfort food speaks to something deeper than hunger – it satisfies emotional needs, connects us to cherished memories, and provides the kind of soul-warming satisfaction that turns a house into a home. Everyone has their favorite comfort food, those dishes that bring instant calm to a chaotic day or celebration to an ordinary evening.

When I received my celiac diagnosis, I grieved the loss of many comforting favorites. I tried reimagining them with disappointing results – gluten-free pasta that never quite had the right texture, bread substitutes that promised but didn't deliver. Then something unexpected happened. My first truly satisfying meal after diagnosis wasn't a reimagined version of something I'd lost – it was something completely new and different: Corn Polenta Rounds with Mushroom Ragout.

I happened to be eating dinner alone, lost in the love of cooking just for myself and able to explore any flavor I wanted. I looked at the items in my fridge and pantry differently as I could just take care of myself for one moment.

I still remember that first bite. The crispy exterior of the pan-seared polenta giving way to creamy, Parmesan-enriched softness. The earthy mushroom ragout, rich with wine and fresh herbs, creating layers of sophisticated yet deeply comforting flavor. It wasn't trying to be something else. It was creative, tasty, balanced – and it became my new favorite comfort food dinner. That meal taught me an invaluable lesson: sometimes the path forward isn't about recreating what we've lost, but discovering what delights us now.

It's perfectly okay to treat your culinary adventure as your personal journey. It’s Ok to to discover and create new comfort foods, even if they are just for you.

These reimagined classics prove that the essence of comfort food lies not in specific ingredients, but in the feelings of warmth, satisfaction, and care that come from lovingly prepared meals. Each recipe maintains the spirit and satisfaction of beloved traditional dishes while incorporating techniques and ingredients that support your health goals. The result is food that comforts both body and soul, creating new traditions that honor the past while embracing a healthier future.

Corn Polenta Rounds with Mushroom Ragout

This was the first dish that I made for myself after my celiac diagnoses that actually felt satisfying. Elegant comfort food that transforms humble cornmeal into sophisticated rounds topped with an earthy, wine-enriched mushroom ragout. This dish bridges rustic Italian tradition with refined presentation, perfect for entertaining or elevating a weeknight dinner.

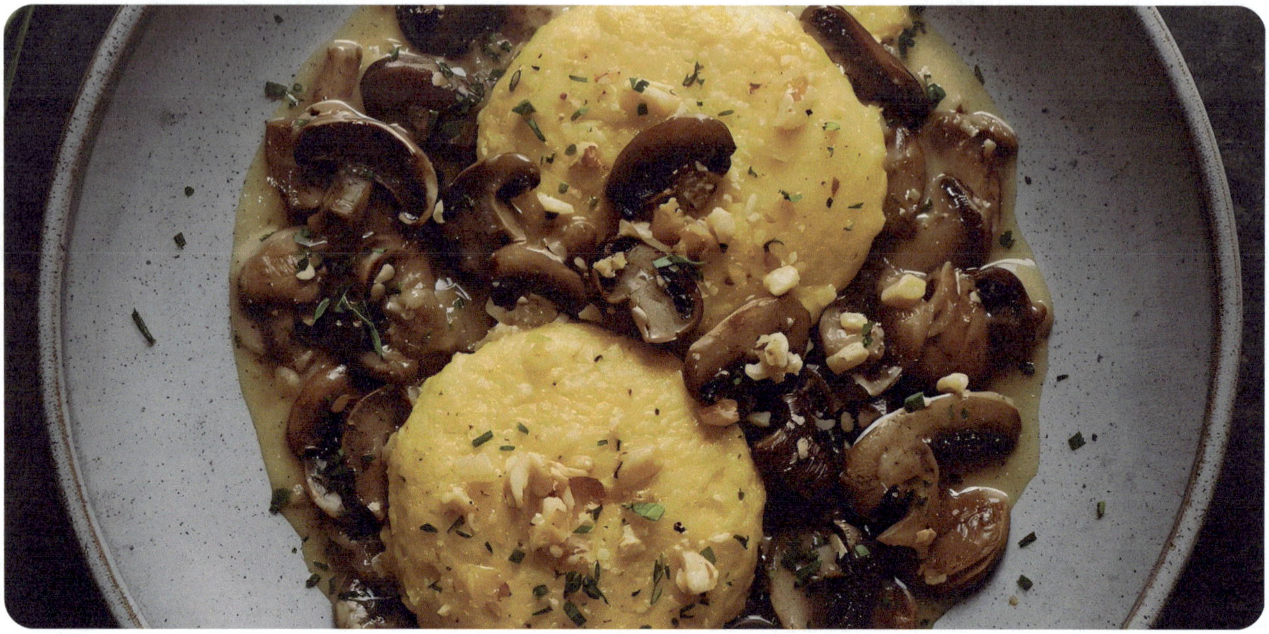

6

30 minutes (plus 2 hours chilling)

45 minutes

INGREDIENTS

For polenta rounds:

- 2 cups coarse polenta (ensure gluten-free)
- 6 cups vegetable broth (low-sodium)
- 1/2 cup whole milk
- 4 tablespoons butter
- 1/2 cup Parmesan cheese, grated
- 2 tablespoons fresh chives, chopped
- 1 teaspoon salt
- 1/4 teaspoon white pepper
- 2 tablespoons olive oil (for pan-searing)

For mushroom ragout:

- 1 lb mixed wild mushrooms (shiitake, cremini, oyster), sliced
- 8 oz baby portobello mushrooms, quartered
- 3 tablespoons olive oil
- 2 shallots, minced
- 4 cloves garlic, minced
- 1/2 cup dry white wine
- 1/4 cup heavy cream
- 2 tablespoons fresh thyme leaves
- 2 tablespoons fresh parsley, chopped
- 1 tablespoon fresh rosemary, minced
- 1 teaspoon truffle oil (optional)
- Salt and black pepper to taste
- 1/4 cup toasted pine nuts for garnish
- Fresh herb sprigs for garnish

DIRECTIONS

Make polenta rounds:

1. Line a 9x13-inch baking dish with parchment paper and lightly oil.
2. In large, heavy-bottomed saucepan, bring vegetable broth to a boil over medium-high heat.
3. Gradually whisk in polenta in a steady stream to prevent lumps. Reduce heat to low.
4. Cook, stirring frequently with wooden spoon, for 25-30 minutes until polenta pulls away from sides of pan and is thick enough to hold its shape.
5. Remove from heat and stir in milk, butter, Parmesan, chives, salt, and white pepper until smooth.
6. Pour polenta into prepared baking dish and smooth top with offset spatula.
7. Cover with plastic wrap, pressing directly onto surface to prevent skin formation. Refrigerate at least 2 hours or overnight until firm.

Prepare mushroom ragout:

1. Heat olive oil in large skillet over medium-high heat.
2. Add mushrooms in single layer (work in batches if necessary) and cook without stirring for 4-5 minutes until golden brown.
3. Stir mushrooms and continue cooking 3-4 minutes until tender and caramelized. Season with salt and pepper.
4. Add shallots and cook 2 minutes until softened. Add garlic and cook 1 minute until fragrant.
5. Pour in white wine and scrape up any browned bits. Let wine reduce by half, about 3 minutes.
6. Lower heat and stir in cream, thyme, parsley, and rosemary. Simmer 2-3 minutes until slightly thickened.
7. Remove from heat and drizzle with truffle oil if using. Adjust seasoning and keep warm.

Assemble and serve:

1. Remove polenta from refrigerator and cut into 12 rounds using 3-inch cookie cutter or glass. (Save scraps for another use.)
2. Heat 2 tablespoons olive oil in large non-stick skillet over medium heat.
3. Pan-sear polenta rounds 3-4 minutes per side until golden brown and heated through. Work in batches if necessary.
4. Arrange 2 polenta rounds on each serving plate.
5. Spoon mushroom ragout generously over and around polenta rounds.
6. Garnish with toasted pine nuts and fresh herb sprigs. Serve immediately.

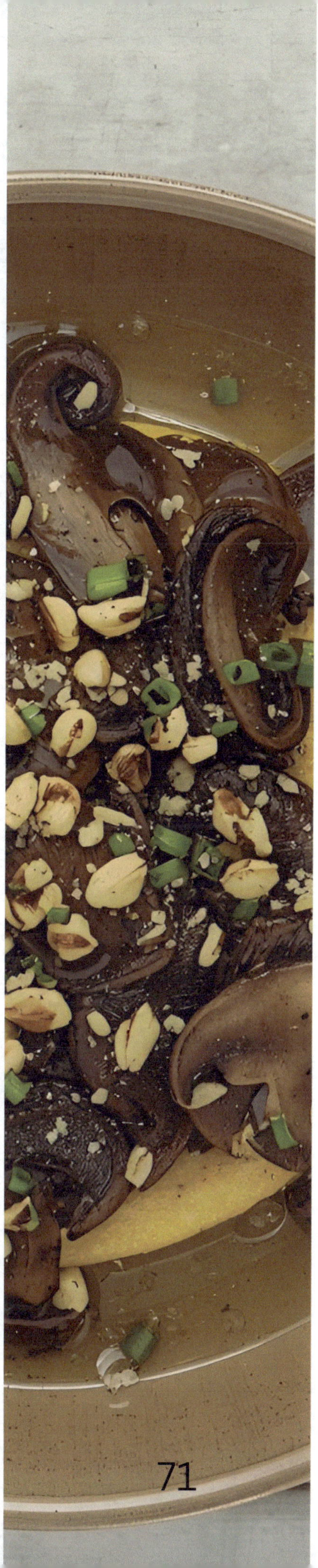

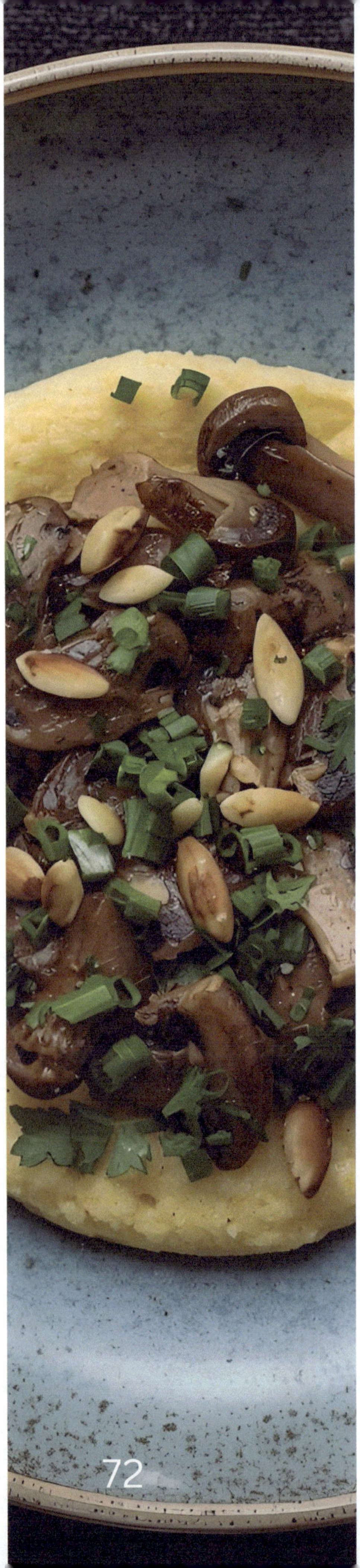

Make-Ahead Tip

Polenta can be made up to 2 days ahead and refrigerated. Mushroom ragout can be prepared 4 hours ahead and reheated gently before serving.

VARIATIONS

- Add 1/4 cup sun-dried tomatoes to ragout for Mediterranean flair
- Substitute goat cheese for Parmesan in polenta for tangier flavor
- Use vegetable broth instead of wine for alcohol-free version

NUTRITION

Per serving: 285 calories, 8g protein, 24g carbohydrates, 18g fat, 4g fiber

STORAGE

Leftover polenta rounds keep for 3 days refrigerated. Reheat in oven at 350°F for 10 minutes. Ragout keeps for 2 days refrigerated.

Herb Crusted "Fried" Chicken

Achieve crispy, golden chicken through oven "frying" with an almond flour and herb coating that rivals any traditional fried chicken.

6 | 20 minutes | 45 minutes

INGREDIENTS

- 3 lbs chicken pieces (thighs, drumsticks, breasts)
- 2 cups almond flour
- 1/2 cup grated Parmesan cheese
- 2 tablespoons dried herbs (rosemary, thyme, oregano)
- 2 teaspoons paprika
- 1 teaspoon garlic powder
- 1 teaspoon onion powder
- 1 teaspoon salt
- 1/2 teaspoon black pepper
- 1/4 teaspoon cayenne pepper
- 3 large eggs, beaten
- 1/4 cup olive oil
- Cooking spray

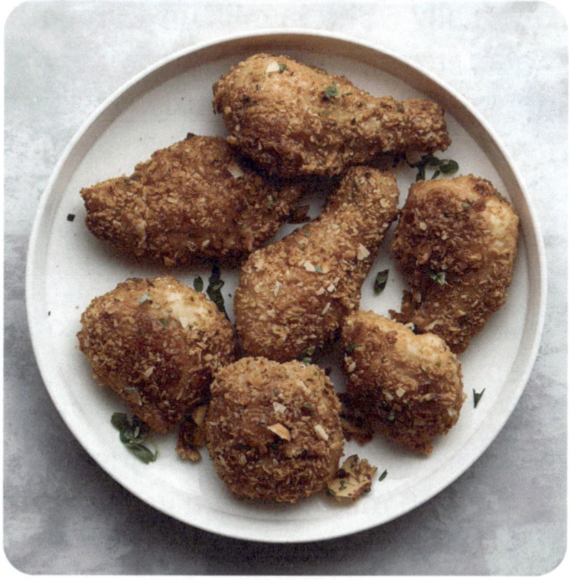

DIRECTIONS

1. Preheat oven to 425°F (220°C). Line large baking sheet with parchment and spray with cooking spray.
2. Pat chicken dry and season with salt and pepper.
3. In shallow dish, combine almond flour, Parmesan, herbs, paprika, garlic powder, onion powder, salt, pepper, and cayenne.
4. In another dish, beat eggs with olive oil.
5. Dip each piece of chicken in egg mixture, then coat thoroughly in almond flour mixture.
6. Place on prepared baking sheet, leaving space between pieces.
7. Spray tops of chicken with cooking spray.
8. Bake 35-45 minutes until coating is golden and internal temperature reaches 165°F (74°C).
9. Let rest 5 minutes before serving.

NUTRITION

Per serving: 485 calories, 42g protein, 8g carbohydrates, 32g fat, 4g fiber

STORAGE

Leftovers keep for up to 3 days refrigerated. Reheat in 375°F oven for 10 minutes to restore crispiness.

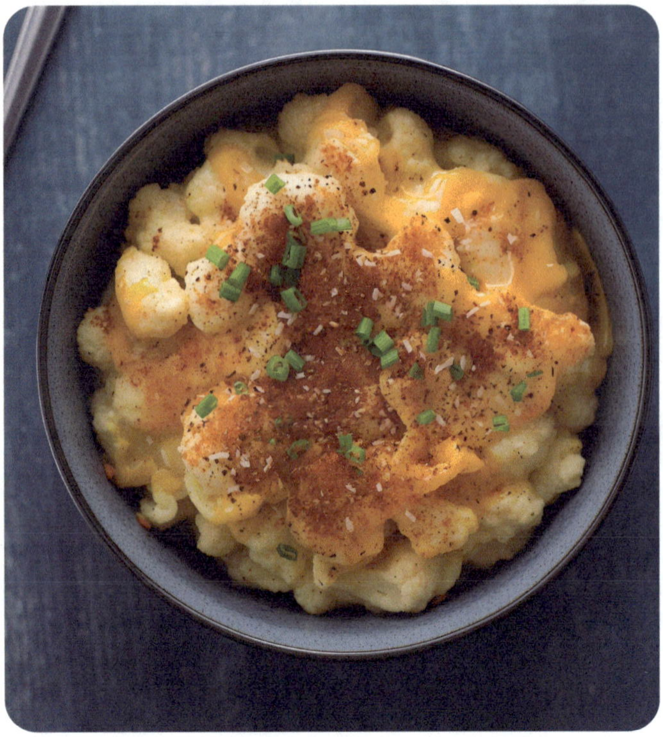

Cauliflower Mac and Cheese

Creamy, cheesy comfort food that substitutes cauliflower for pasta while maintaining all the rich satisfaction of the original.

8	20 minutes	35 minutes

NUTRITION

Per serving: 285 calories, 16g protein, 12g carbohydrates, 21g fat, 4g fiber

STORAGE

Can be assembled 1 day ahead. Refrigerate covered, then bake as directed, adding 10 minutes to cooking time.

INGREDIENTS

- 2 large heads cauliflower, cut into florets
- 4 tablespoons butter
- 1/4 cup almond flour
- 2 cups whole milk
- 2 cups sharp cheddar cheese, shredded
- 1/2 cup cream cheese, softened
- 1/4 cup Parmesan cheese, grated
- 1 teaspoon Dijon mustard
- 1/2 teaspoon garlic powder
- 1/2 teaspoon salt
- 1/4 teaspoon black pepper
- 1/4 teaspoon paprika
- 2 tablespoons fresh chives, chopped

DIRECTION

1. Preheat oven to 375°F (190°C). Grease 9x13-inch baking dish.
2. In a large pot steam cauliflower florets until just tender, about 8 minutes. Drain well.
3. In large saucepan, melt butter over medium heat. Whisk in almond flour and cook 2 minutes.
4. Gradually whisk in milk until smooth. Cook, stirring constantly, until thickened, about 5 minutes.
5. Remove from heat and stir in cheddar cheese, cream cheese, Parmesan, Dijon mustard, garlic powder, salt, and pepper until smooth.
6. Fold in cauliflower and transfer to prepared baking dish.
7. Sprinkle with paprika and bake 25 minutes until bubbly and golden.
8. Let rest 10 minutes, then garnish with chives before serving.

Meatloaf with Mushroom Gravy

Classic comfort food elevated with Mediterranean flavors that add depth and sophistication while maintaining familiar appeal.

8 | 20 minutes | 1 hour

INGREDIENTS

For meatloaf:

- 2 lbs ground beef (85/15)
- 1 cup almond flour
- 1/2 cup sun-dried tomatoes (oil packed), chopped
- 1/4 cup fresh basil, chopped
- 1 large onion, finely diced
- 2 cloves garlic, minced
- 2 large eggs
- 1/4 cup milk
- 2 tablespoons balsamic vinegar
- 1 teaspoon salt
- 1/2 teaspoon black pepper

For mushroom gravy:

- 2 tablespoons butter
- 8 oz mushrooms, sliced
- 2 tablespoons almond flour
- 2 cups low sodium beef broth
- 2 tablespoons heavy cream
- Salt and pepper to taste

For glaze:

- 3 tablespoons balsamic vinegar
- 2 tablespoons honey
- 1 tablespoon Dijon mustard

NUTRITION

Per serving: 365 calories, 28g protein, 10g carbohydrates, 24g fat, 3g fiber

STORAGE

Meatloaf keeps for up to 4 days refrigerated or 3 months frozen.

DIRECTIONS

1. Preheat oven to 375°F (190°C). Line loaf pan with parchment paper.
2. In large bowl, combine ground beef, almond flour, sun-dried tomatoes, basil, onion, garlic, eggs, milk, balsamic vinegar, salt, and pepper. Mix gently until just combined.
3. Shape into loaf and place in prepared pan.
4. Make glaze: Whisk together balsamic vinegar, honey, and Dijon mustard. Brush over meatloaf.
5. Bake 50-60 minutes until internal temperature reaches 160°F (71°C).
6. Make gravy: In large skillet, melt butter and sauté mushrooms until golden. Sprinkle with almond flour and cook 2 minutes. Gradually add broth, stirring until thickened. Stir in cream and season.
7. Let meatloaf rest 10 minutes before slicing. Serve with mushroom gravy.

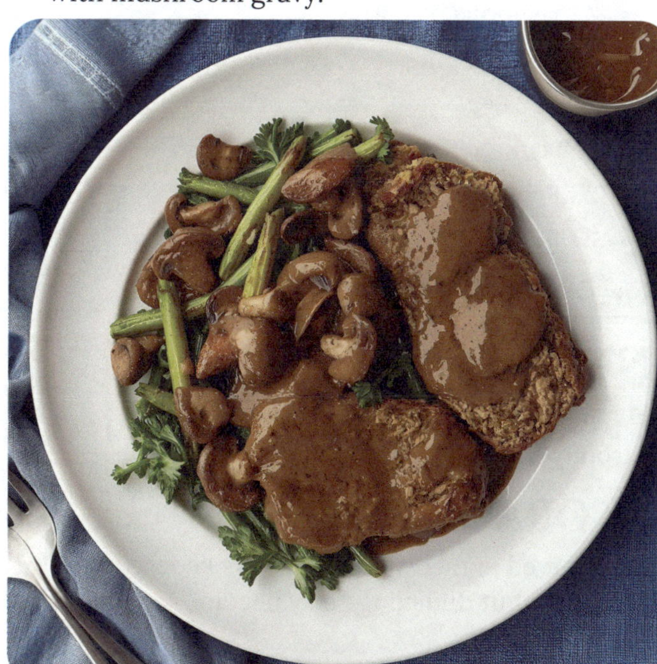

Chicken and Dumplings

Servings	Prep time	Cook time
6	30 minutes	45 minutes

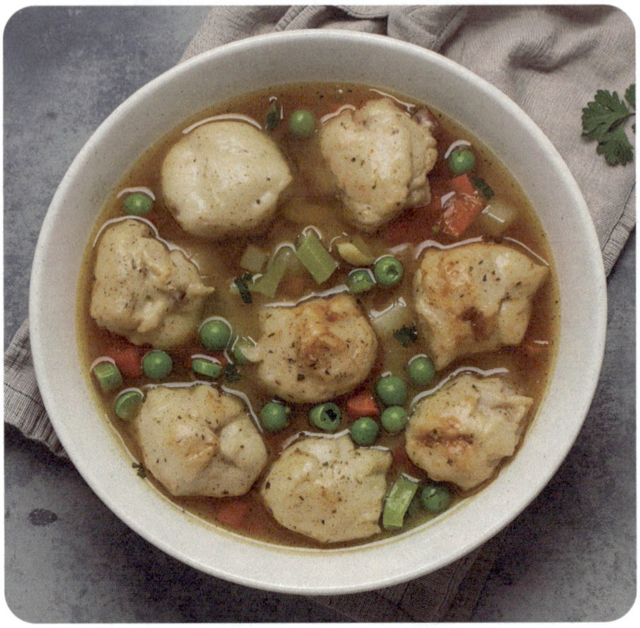

Fluffy almond flour dumplings float in a rich chicken stew, creating the ultimate one-pot comfort meal.

INGREDIENTS

For stew:

- 2 lbs chicken thighs, boneless and skinless, cut into chunks
- 2 tablespoons olive oil
- 1 large onion, diced
- 3 carrots, sliced
- 3 celery stalks, diced
- 3 cloves garlic, minced
- 6 cups low sodium chicken broth
- 2 bay leaves
- 1 teaspoon dried thyme
- 1 cup frozen peas
- Salt and pepper to taste

For dumplings:

- 1 1/2 cups almond flour
- 1/2 cup tapioca starch
- 2 teaspoons baking powder
- 1 teaspoon salt
- 2 large eggs
- 1/2 cup milk
- 2 tablespoons melted butter
- 2 tablespoons fresh parsley, chopped

NUTRITION

Per serving: 425 calories, 35g protein, 18g carbohydrates, 25g fat, 4g fiber

STORAGE

Best served immediately. Leftovers keep for 2 days but dumplings may become soft.

DIRECTIONS

1. Heat olive oil in large Dutch oven over medium-high heat. Season chicken and brown on all sides, about 8 minutes. Remove and set aside.
2. Add onion, carrots, and celery to same pot. Cook 8 minutes until softened.
3. Add garlic and cook 1 minute until fragrant.
4. Return chicken to pot with broth, bay leaves, and thyme. Bring to boil, then simmer 20 minutes.
5. Make dumplings: In bowl, whisk together almond flour, tapioca starch, baking powder, and salt. In another bowl, whisk eggs, milk, melted butter, and parsley. Combine wet and dry ingredients until just mixed.
6. Remove bay leaves from stew. Add peas and bring to gentle boil.
7. Drop dumpling batter by spoonfuls into simmering stew. Cover and cook 15 minutes without lifting lid.
8. Season with salt and pepper before serving.

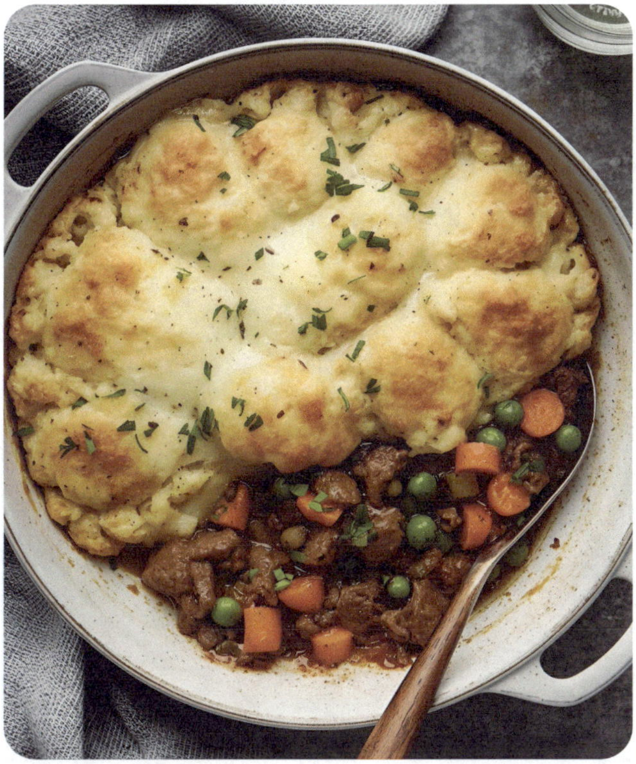

Shepherd's Pie with Cauliflower Mash

8 | 30 minutes | 45 minutes

A hearty, layered casserole topped with creamy cauliflower mash instead of potatoes for a lighter but equally satisfying version.

INGREDIENTS

For filling:

- 2 lbs ground lamb or beef
- 1 large onion, diced
- 2 carrots, diced
- 2 celery stalks, diced
- 3 cloves garlic, minced
- 2 tablespoons tomato paste
- 1 cup red wine (optional) or additional broth
- 2 cups beef broth
- 2 tablespoons fresh rosemary, chopped
- 1 tablespoon fresh thyme
- 1 cup frozen peas
- Salt and pepper to taste

For cauliflower mash:

- 2 large heads cauliflower, cut into florets
- 4 tablespoons butter
- 1/4 cup heavy cream
- 1/2 cup Parmesan cheese, grated
- Salt and pepper to taste

DIRECTIONS

1. Preheat oven to 400°F (200°C).
2. Make cauliflower mash: In a large pot steam cauliflower until very tender, about 15 minutes. Drain well and mash with butter, cream, and Parmesan. Season with salt and pepper.
3. Make filling: In large skillet, brown ground meat, breaking up with spoon. Remove and drain excess fat.
4. Add onion, carrots, and celery to same pan. Cook 8 minutes until softened.
5. Add garlic and tomato paste, cooking 2 minutes until fragrant.
6. Add wine (if using) and cook until reduced by half. Add broth, rosemary, thyme, and browned meat.
7. Simmer 15 minutes until slightly thickened. Stir in peas and season.
8. Transfer filling to 9x13-inch baking dish. Top with cauliflower mash, spreading evenly.
9. Bake 25-30 minutes until top is golden and filling is bubbling.
10. Let rest 10 minutes before serving.

NUTRITION

Per serving: 385 calories, 28g protein, 12g carbohydrates, 25g fat, 4g fiber

STORAGE

Can be assembled 1 day ahead. Freeze for up to 3 months.

Chicken Pot Pie with Almond Flour Crust

Traditional comfort elevated with sophisticated flavors that add elegance while maintaining the homey appeal of chicken pot pie.

INGREDIENTS

For almond flour crust:

- 2 1/2 cups almond flour
- 1/2 cup tapioca starch
- 1 teaspoon salt
- 1/2 cup cold butter, cubed
- 1 large egg
- 2-3 tablespoons ice water

For filling:

- 3 cups cooked chicken, diced
- 3 tablespoons butter
- 2 large leeks, white parts only, sliced
- 2 carrots, diced
- 2 celery stalks, diced
- 3 cloves garlic, minced
- 1/4 cup almond flour
- 2 cups chicken broth
- 1/2 cup heavy cream
- 1/4 cup white wine
- 2 tablespoons fresh tarragon, chopped
- 1 cup frozen peas
- Salt and pepper to taste
- 1 egg, beaten (for wash)

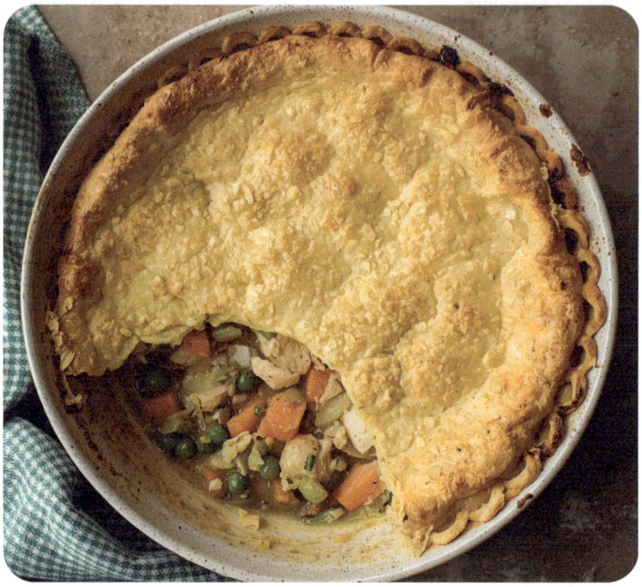

8	45 minutes	40 minutes

DIRECTIONS

1. Make crust: Combine almond flour, tapioca starch, and salt. Cut in cold butter until mixture resembles coarse crumbs. Add egg and ice water gradually until dough forms. Divide in half, wrap, and chill 30 minutes.
2. Preheat oven to 425°F (220°C).
3. Make filling: In large skillet, melt butter and sauté leeks, carrots, and celery until softened, about 8 minutes. Add garlic and cook 1 minute.
4. Sprinkle with almond flour and cook 2 minutes. Gradually add broth, cream, and wine, stirring until thickened.
5. Add chicken, tarragon, and peas. Season with salt and pepper.
6. Sprinkle a cutting board with almond flour and roll out half the dough and place in 9-inch pie pan. Add filling.
7. Roll out remaining dough for top crust. Place over filling and seal edges.
8. Cut vents and brush with beaten egg.
9. Bake 35-40 minutes until crust is golden brown.
10. Let rest 10 minutes before serving.

NUTRITION

Per serving: 465 calories, 25g protein, 16g carbohydrates, 35g fat, 5g fiber

STORAGE

Can be assembled and frozen unbaked for up to 3 months. Bake from frozen, adding 15 minutes to cooking time

Servings	Prep time	Cook time
6	20 minutes	30 minutes

Tuna Noodle Casserole with Shiitake Mushrooms

A sophisticated update to the classic casserole using shiitaki mushrooms and fresh herbs for deeper, more complex flavors.

INGREDIENTS

- 12 oz gluten-free pasta
- 2 cans (5 oz each) tuna in water, drained
- 3 tablespoons butter
- 8 oz shiitaki mushrooms, stems removed, sliced
- 1 medium onion, diced
- 3 cloves garlic, minced
- 1/4 cup almond flour
- 2 cups milk
- 1 cup frozen peas
- 1/2 cup Parmesan cheese, grated
- 2 tablespoons fresh parsley, chopped
- 1 tablespoon fresh thyme
- 1/2 cup almond flour mixed with 2 tablespoons melted butter (for topping)
- Salt and pepper to taste

NUTRITION

Per serving: 385 calories, 24g protein, 45g carbohydrates, 12g fat, 4g fiber

STORAGE

Can be assembled 1 day ahead. Cover and refrigerate, then bake as directed.

DIRECTIONS

1. Preheat oven to 375°F (190°C). Grease 9x13-inch baking dish.
2. Cook pasta according to package directions until just shy of al dente. Drain.
3. In large skillet, melt butter and sauté mushrooms until golden, about 6 minutes. Remove and set aside.
4. In same pan, cook onion until softened, about 5 minutes. Add garlic and cook 1 minute.
5. Sprinkle with almond flour and cook 2 minutes, stirring constantly.
6. Gradually whisk in milk until smooth and thickened, about 5 minutes.
7. Stir in tuna, mushrooms, peas, Parmesan, parsley, and thyme. Season with salt and pepper.
8. Combine pasta with tuna mixture and transfer to prepared baking dish.
9. Top with almond flour-butter mixture.
10. Bake 25 minutes until bubbly and golden on top.

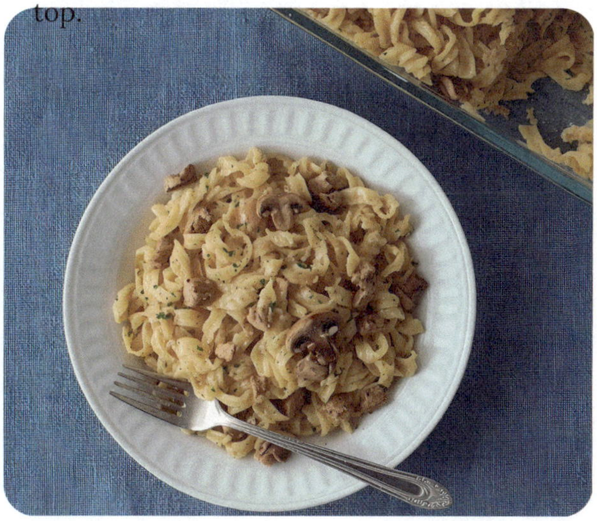

Meatballs in Marinara Sauce

Tender, flavorful meatballs in rich marinara sauce that can be served over zucchini noodles, gluten-free pasta, or on their own.

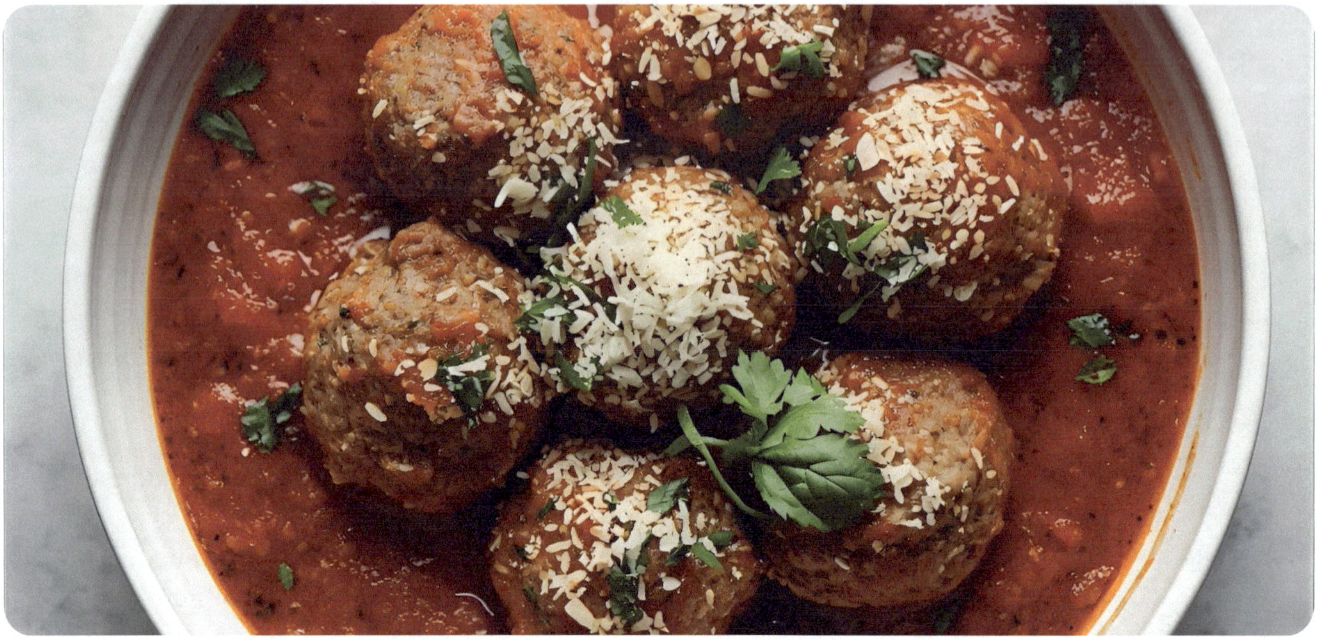

Servings	Prep time	Cook time
6	25 minutes	35 minutes

INGREDIENTS

For meatballs:

- 1 lb ground beef (80/20)
- 1/2 lb ground pork
- 1/2 cup almond flour
- 1/4 cup Parmesan cheese, grated
- 1 large egg
- 1/4 cup milk
- 2 cloves garlic, minced
- 2 tablespoons fresh parsley, chopped
- 1 teaspoon salt
- 1/2 teaspoon black pepper
- 2 tablespoons olive oil

For marinara sauce:

- 2 tablespoons olive oil
- 1 medium onion, diced
- 4 cloves garlic, minced
- 1 can (28 oz) crushed tomatoes
- 1 can (14 oz) diced tomatoes
- 2 tablespoons tomato paste
- 1/4 cup fresh basil, chopped
- 2 teaspoons dried oregano
- 1 teaspoon salt
- 1/2 teaspoon black pepper
- 1 teaspoon sugar (optional)

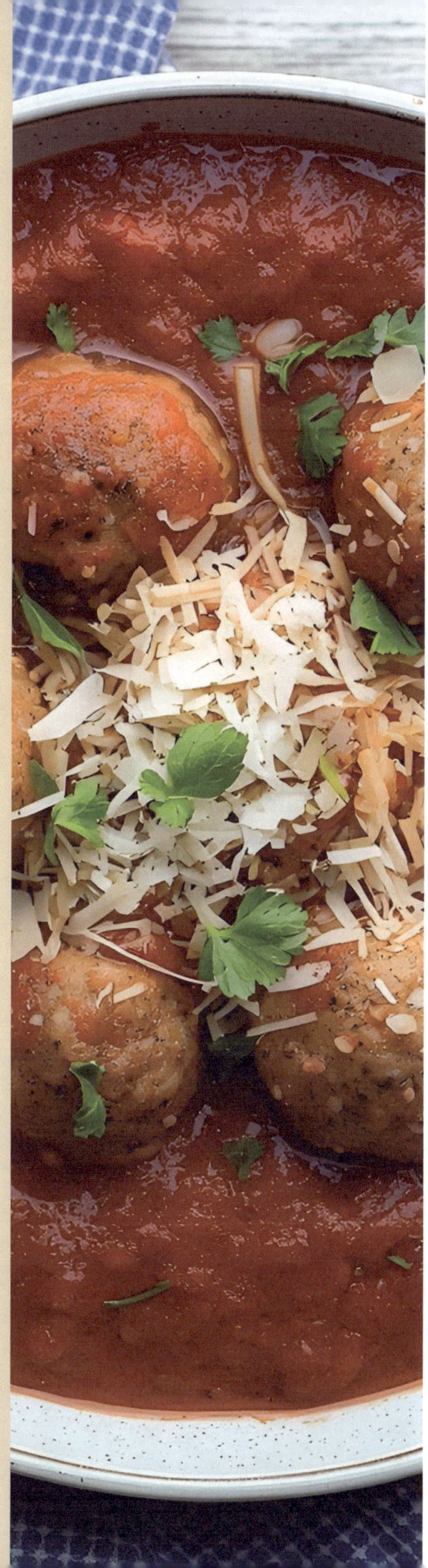

DIRECTIONS

1. Make sauce: Heat olive oil in large pot over medium heat. Cook onion until softened, about 6 minutes. Add garlic and cook 1 minute.
2. Add crushed tomatoes, diced tomatoes, tomato paste, basil, oregano, salt, pepper, and sugar if using. Simmer 20 minutes, stirring occasionally.
3. Make meatballs: In large bowl, combine ground beef, ground pork, almond flour, Parmesan, egg, milk, garlic, parsley, salt, and pepper. Mix gently until just combined.
4. Roll into 24 meatballs, about 1.5 inches diameter.
5. Heat olive oil in large skillet over medium-high heat. Brown meatballs in batches, turning to brown all sides, about 8 minutes total.
6. Add browned meatballs to marinara sauce and simmer 15 minutes until cooked through.
7. Serve hot over desired base, garnished with additional basil and Parmesan.

NUTRITION

Per serving: 4 meatballs with sauce: 345 calories, 25g protein, 12g carbohydrates, 22g fat, 3g fiber

STORAGE

Meatballs and sauce freeze beautifully for up to 3 months. Thaw overnight and reheat gently.

Chicken Parmesan with Zucchini

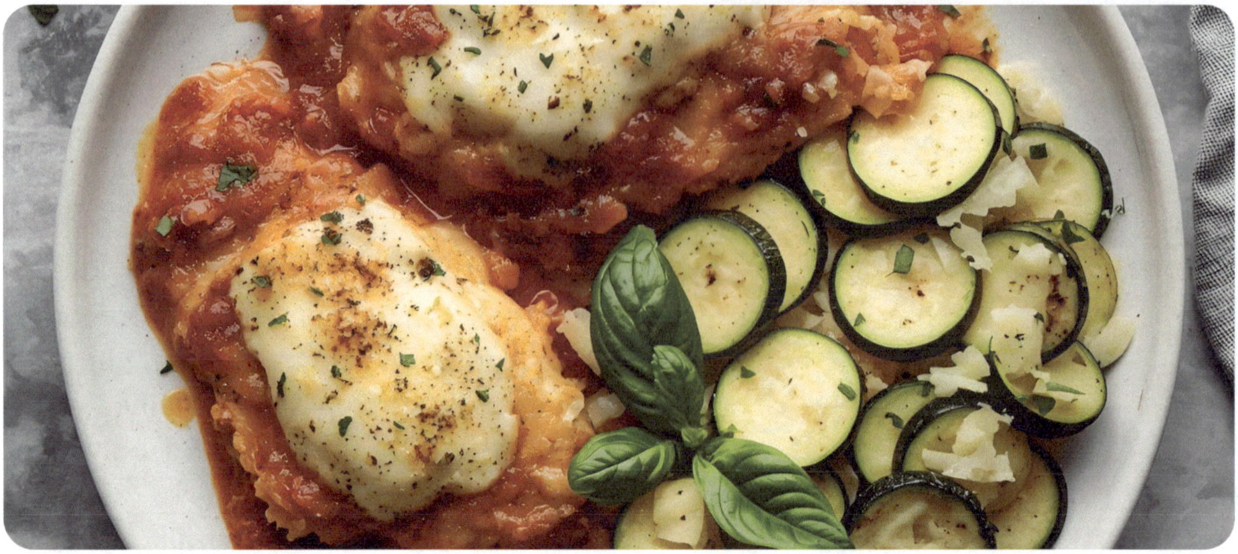

INGREDIENTS

- 6 boneless, skinless chicken breasts, pounded to 1/2-inch thickness
- 1 1/2 cups almond flour
- 1/2 cup Parmesan cheese, grated
- 2 teaspoons Italian seasoning
- 1 teaspoon garlic powder
- 1 teaspoon salt
- 1/2 teaspoon black pepper
- 3 large eggs, beaten
- 1/4 cup olive oil
- 2 cups marinara sauce (from previous recipe or store-bought)
- 1 1/2 cups mozzarella cheese, shredded
- 1/4 cup fresh basil, chopped
- 4 medium zucchini, sliced lengthwise into planks
- 2 tablespoons olive oil for zucchini

NUTRITION

Per serving: 485 calories, 45g protein, 14g carbohydrates, 28g fat, 5g fiber

STORAGE

Breaded chicken can be cooked 1 day ahead. Assemble and bake when ready to serve.

Crispy breaded chicken topped with marinara and melted cheese, served alongside roasted zucchini for a complete, satisfying meal.

6 | 25 minutes | 35 minutes

DIRECTIONS

1. Preheat oven to 425°F (220°C).
2. In shallow dish, combine almond flour, Parmesan, Italian seasoning, garlic powder, salt, and pepper.
3. Dip each chicken breast in beaten eggs, then coat thoroughly in almond flour mixture.
4. Heat olive oil in large oven-safe skillet over medium-high heat. Brown chicken 3-4 minutes per side until golden.
5. Meanwhile, toss zucchini planks with olive oil, salt, and pepper. Arrange on baking sheet.
6. Top each chicken breast with marinara sauce and mozzarella cheese.
7. Place chicken skillet and zucchini in oven. Bake 15-20 minutes until chicken reaches 165°F (74°C) and zucchini is tender.
8. Garnish with fresh basil before serving.

Black Bean & Quinoa Stuffed Peppers

INGREDIENTS

- 6 large bell peppers, tops cut off, seeded
- 1 cup quinoa, rinsed
- 1.5 cups vegetable broth
- 1 can (15 oz) black beans, rinsed
- 1 cup corn kernels (fresh or frozen)
- 1 small onion, diced
- 2 cloves garlic, minced
- 1 tsp chili powder
- ½ tsp cumin
- Salt and black pepper to taste
- ½ cup grated cheddar cheese (optional)
- ¼ cup chopped cilantro

6	20 minutes	30 minutes

Colorful bell peppers stuffed with a hearty mix of quinoa, beans, and spices.

DIRECTIONS

1. Preheat oven to 375°F (190°C).
2. Cook quinoa in broth according to package directions.
3. Sauté onion and garlic until soft. Add black beans, corn, chili powder, cumin, salt, and pepper. Stir in quinoa.
4. Stuff peppers with filling, top with cheese if using, and bake 25–30 min until peppers are tender.
5. Garnish with cilantro before serving.

NUTRITION

Per serving without cheese: 220 calories, 9g protein, 42g carbohydrates, 2g fat, 8g fiber

STORAGE

Keeps refrigerated for up to 5 days. Freezes well (3 months).

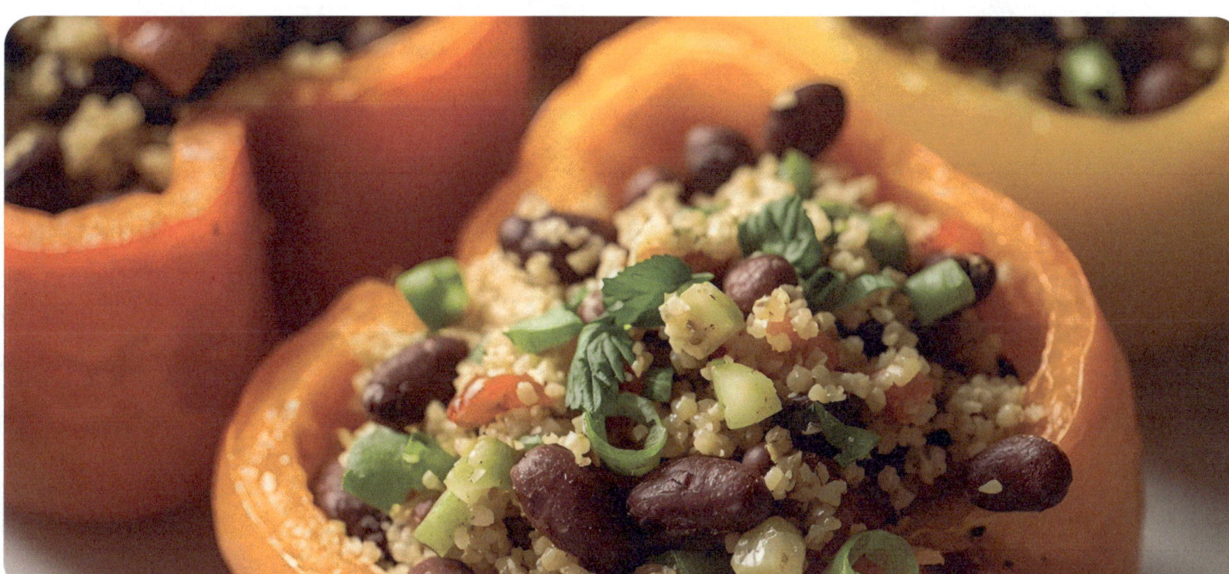

6

15 minutes

45 minutes

Maple Roasted Pork Tenderloin with Brussel Sprouts & Apples

Tender pork roasted with caramelized Brussels sprouts and sweet apples in cider-maple glaze.

INGREDIENTS

- 2 pork tenderloins (about 1 lb each)
- 1 lb brussels sprouts, halved
- 2 apples, cored and sliced
- 3 tbsp olive oil
- ¼ cup apple cider
- 1 tbsp sugar free maple syrup
- 2 cloves garlic, minced
- 1 tsp Dijon mustard
- 1 tsp fresh thyme leaves
- Salt and black pepper to taste

NUTRITION

Per serving: 310 calories, 32g protein, 22g carbohydrates, 11g fat, 5g fiber

STORAGE

Keeps refrigerated for up to 4 days.

DIRECTIONS

1. Preheat oven to 400°F (200°C).
2. Toss Brussels sprouts and apples with 1 tbsp olive oil, salt, and pepper. Spread on a sheet pan.
3. In a bowl, whisk cider, maple syrup, garlic, mustard, thyme, remaining oil, salt, and pepper.
4. Place pork on pan. Brush with half the cider mixture.
5. Roast 20 min, then brush with remaining mixture and roast 20–25 min more, until pork is cooked through and vegetables are caramelized.
6. Let pork rest 5 min before slicing.

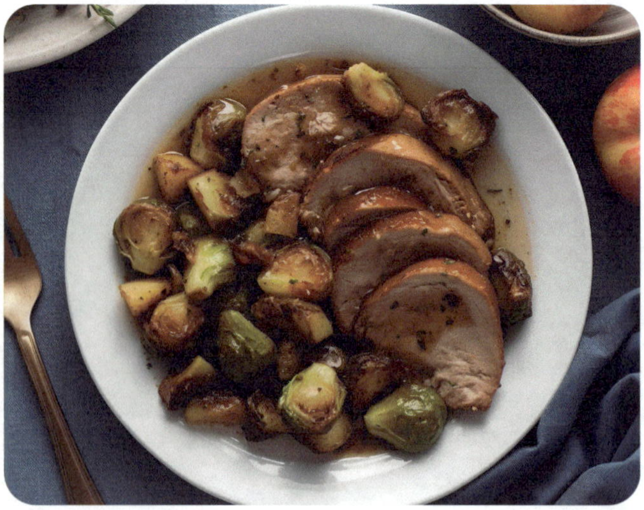

Herb-Grilled Flank Steak with Wilted Greens

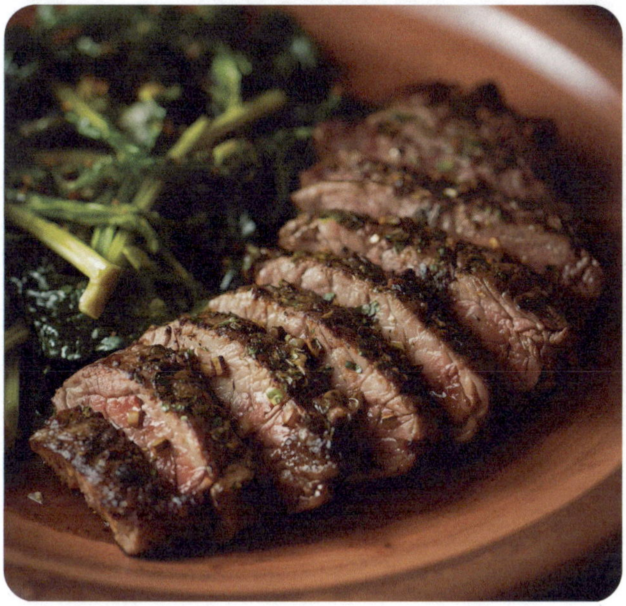

Servings	Prep Time	Cook Time	Rest Time
4	20 minutes	15 minutes	Rest Time

Lean flank steak meets a bright herb marinade and quick-sautéed greens for a balanced, weeknight-friendly meal that feels restaurant special.

INGREDIENTS

- 1½ lbs flank steak
- 3 tbsp olive oil, divided
- 2 tbsp lemon juice
- 3 cloves garlic, minced
- ¼ cup chopped parsley
- 2 tbsp chopped cilantro or basil
- 1 tsp Dijon mustard
- Salt & pepper to taste
- 1 bunch kale or spinach, roughly chopped

DIRECTIONS

1. Marinate Steak: In a small bowl, whisk 2 tbsp olive oil, lemon juice, garlic, herbs, mustard, salt, and pepper. Rub over steak; marinate 20–30 minutes.
2. Grill: Heat grill or grill pan over medium-high. Cook steak 4–5 minutes per side for medium-rare. Rest 5 minutes before slicing thinly against the grain.
3. Wilt Greens: In a skillet, heat 1 tbsp olive oil. Add greens and sauté 2–3 minutes until just wilted. Season lightly with salt and pepper.
4. Serve: Layer steak slices over greens and drizzle any pan juices on top.

NUTRITION

Per serving, 340 calories, 31g protein, 5g carbohydrates, 22g fat, 2g fiber

STORAGE

Leftovers store for up to 3 days and make a great base for other recipes.

Asian-Glazed Beef Skewers

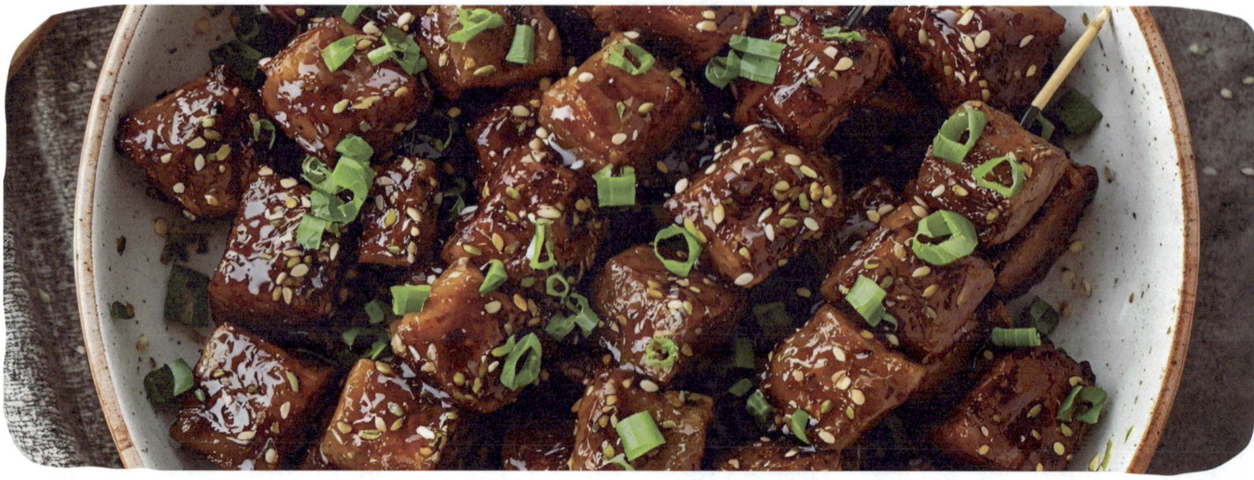

INGREDIENTS

- 2 lbs beef sirloin, cut into 1-inch cubes
- 1/4 cup low-sodium soy sauce (gluten-free)
- 3 tablespoons honey
- 2 tablespoons rice vinegar
- 1 tablespoon sesame oil
- 3 cloves garlic, minced
- 1 tablespoon fresh ginger, minced
- 1/4 teaspoon red pepper flakes
- 2 green onions, sliced
- 1 tablespoon sesame seeds
- Wooden skewers, soaked 30 minutes

NUTRITION

Per serving: 245 calories, 28g protein, 8g carbohydrates, 10g fat, 0g fiber

STORAGE

Best served immediately. Can be assembled and marinated 1 day ahead.

6	20 minutes (Plus 2 hours marinating)	10 minutes	5 minutes

Tender beef with a sweet-savory glaze that caramelizes beautifully on the grill.

DIRECTIONS

Outdoor Grill Method:

1. Combine soy sauce, honey, rice vinegar, sesame oil, garlic, ginger, and red pepper flakes.
2. Marinate beef cubes 2-8 hours in refrigerator.
3. Thread beef onto skewers, reserving marinade.
4. Preheat grill to medium-high heat (400°F/200°C).
5. Grill skewers 8-10 minutes, turning every 2 minutes and basting with reserved marinade.
6. Rest skewers 5 minutes before serving.
7. Garnish with green onions and sesame seeds.

Indoor Alternatives:

1. **Grill Pan:** Cook in batches, 2-3 minutes per side.
2. **Broiler:** Broil 4 inches from element, 8-10 minutes total, turning once.

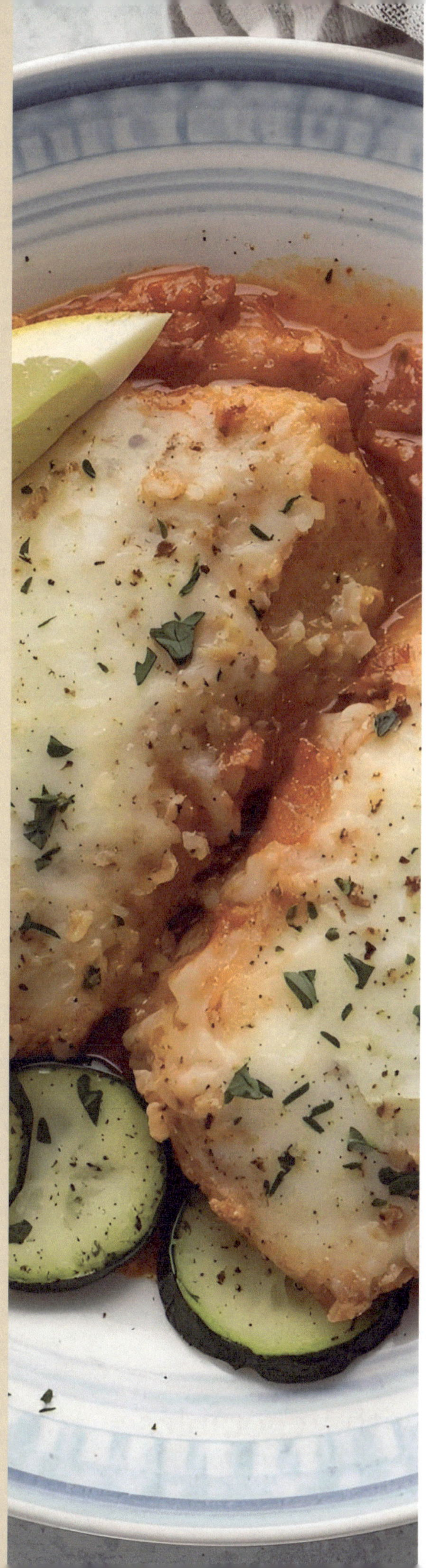

TIPS FOR PERFECT SUCCESSFUL COMFORT FOOD REIMAGINING

Respect the Original: The best reimagined recipes maintain the essence and satisfaction of the original while adapting techniques and ingredients. Focus on preserving textures, flavors, and the emotional satisfaction that makes comfort food special.

Build Flavor Layers: Comfort food relies on deep, developed flavors. Take time to properly brown meats, sauté aromatics, and allow sauces to reduce. These steps create the richness that defines satisfying comfort meals.

Portion Awareness: Comfort foods can be calorie-dense. Balance richer main dishes with lighter sides, and remember that satisfaction often comes from quality rather than quantity.

Seasonal Adaptations: Many comfort foods work beautifully with seasonal ingredient swaps - root vegetables in winter, fresh herbs and lighter preparations in summer.

Remember that the goal isn't to create perfect replicas of traditional dishes, but to capture their spirit and satisfaction while supporting your health goals. The best reimagined comfort foods become new family favorites that happen to be healthier, rather than diet versions of beloved classics.

CHAPTER 08

One-Pan Wonders

The beauty of one-pan cooking lies not just in the minimal cleanup, but in the way flavors meld and intensify when ingredients cook together. These recipes prove that simplicity doesn't mean sacrificing complexity or satisfaction. Each dish is carefully orchestrated so that proteins, vegetables, and seasonings cook at the proper pace, creating complete, balanced meals from a single vessel. Whether you're cooking for busy weeknights or leisurely weekends, these recipes deliver maximum flavor with minimum fuss, leaving you more time to enjoy the meal and the company.

List of Recipes

6 | 15 minutes | 35 minutes

Mediterranean Chicken and Vegetables

Chicken thighs, bell peppers, zucchini, and cherry tomatoes roast together with herbs and lemon for a vibrant, healthy dinner.

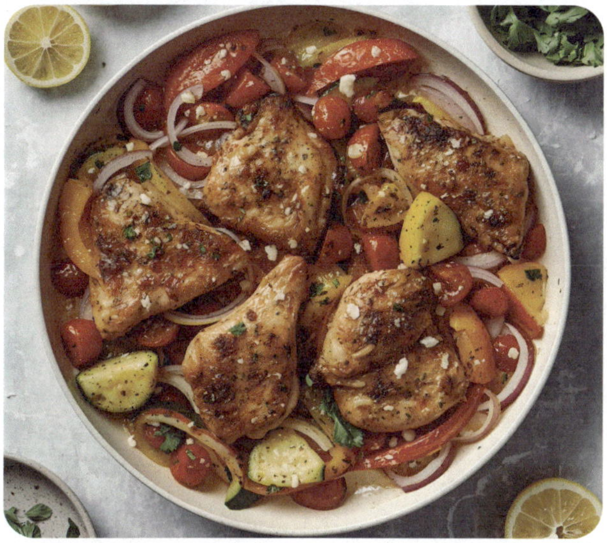

INGREDIENTS

- 8 bone-in, skin-on chicken thighs
- 2 red bell peppers, cut into strips
- 2 yellow bell peppers, cut into strips
- 2 medium zucchini, sliced into half-moons
- 1 pint cherry tomatoes
- 1 red onion, cut into wedges
- 1/4 cup olive oil
- 3 cloves garlic, minced
- 2 tablespoons fresh oregano (or 2 teaspoons dried)
- 1 tablespoon fresh thyme
- 1 lemon, juiced and zested
- 1/2 cup Kalamata olives, pitted
- 1/4 cup fresh parsley, chopped
- Salt and black pepper to taste

NUTRITION

Per serving: 385 calories, 28g protein, 12g carbohydrates, 26g fat, 3g fiber

STORAGE

Leftovers keep for up to 3 days refrigerated. Reheat in 350°F oven for 15 minutes.

DIRECTIONS

1. Preheat oven to 425°F (220°C).
2. Pat chicken thighs dry and season generously with salt and pepper.
3. In large bowl, toss bell peppers, zucchini, cherry tomatoes, and red onion with olive oil, garlic, oregano, thyme, lemon zest, salt, and pepper.
4. Arrange vegetables on large rimmed baking sheet. Nestle chicken thighs among vegetables, skin side up.
5. Roast 30-35 minutes until chicken skin is golden and internal temperature reaches 165°F (74°C).
6. Add olives during last 5 minutes of cooking.
7. Drizzle with lemon juice and sprinkle with fresh parsley before serving.

6

15 minutes

35 minutes

Chipotle Chickpea & Sweet Potato Skillet

Smoky chipotle chickpeas and sweet potatoes simmered into a hearty one-pan meal.

INGREDIENTS

- 2 large sweet potatoes, diced
- 2 cans (15 oz each) chickpeas, rinsed
- 1 bell pepper, diced
- 1 can (14.5 oz) fire-roasted tomatoes
- 2 cloves garlic, minced
- 1 tbsp chipotle in adobo, minced
- 1 tsp smoked paprika
- Salt and black pepper to taste
- 2 tbsp olive oil
- Lime wedges and avocado for serving

DIRECTIONS

1. Heat oil in a large skillet. Add sweet potatoes and pepper; cook 10 min until softened.
2. Add garlic, chipotle, paprika, salt, and pepper; stir 1 min.
3. Stir in tomatoes and chickpeas.
4. Cover and simmer 20 min until sweet potatoes are tender.
5. Top with lime wedges and avocado slices.

NUTRITION

Per serving: 280 calories, 10g protein, 45g carbohydrates, 8g fat, 10g fiber

STORAGE

Keeps 5 days refrigerated.

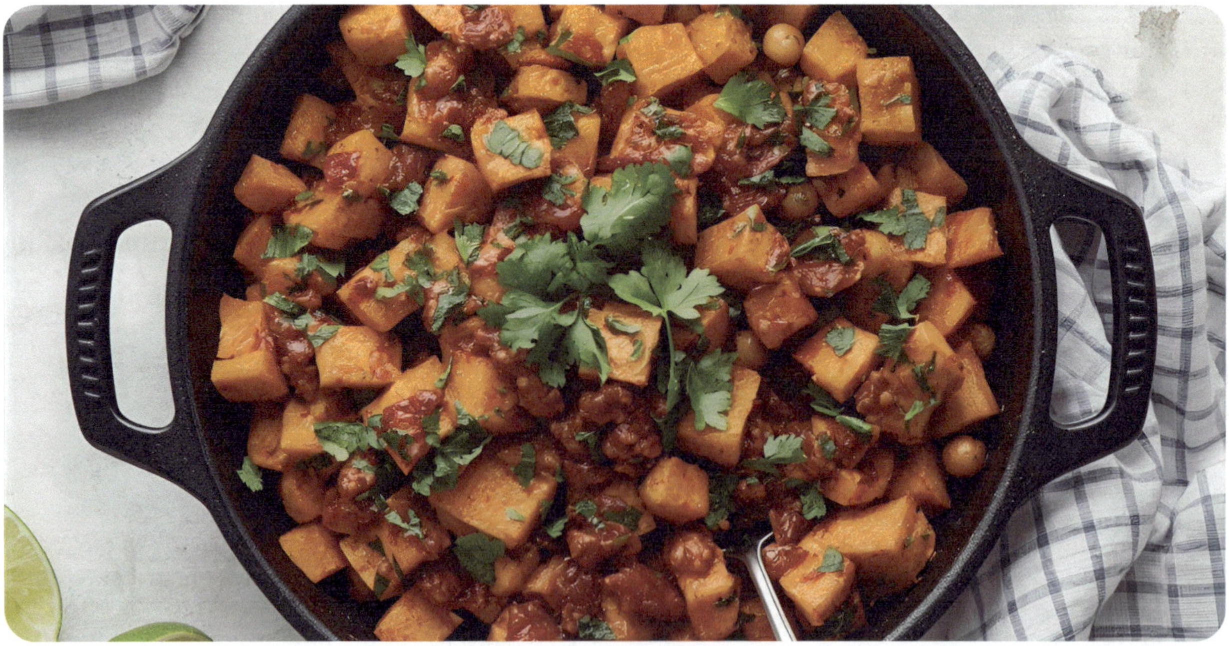

Lemon Herb Salmon with Asparagus

Servings	Prep time	Cook time
4	10 minutes	15 minutes

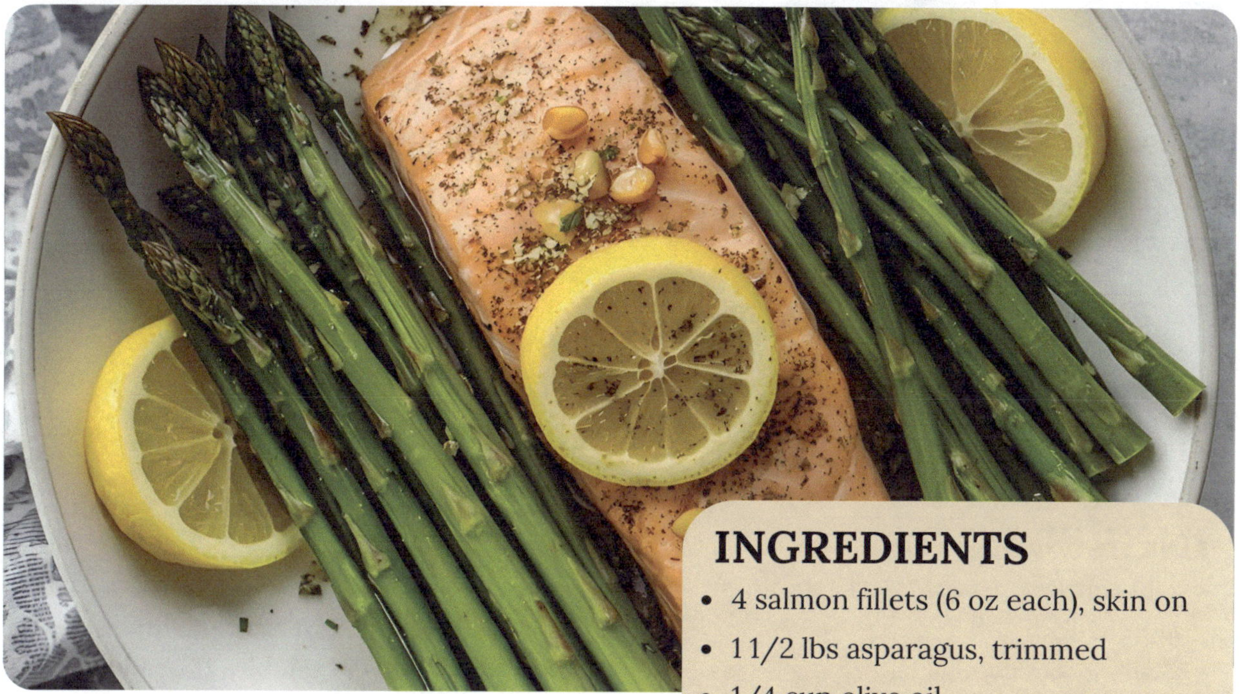

Elegant salmon enhanced with the bright, salty intensity of preserved lemons and the unexpected coolness of fresh mint and crunchy pistachios.

INGREDIENTS

- 4 salmon fillets (6 oz each), skin on
- 1 1/2 lbs asparagus, trimmed
- 1/4 cup olive oil
- 2 preserved lemons, rinsed and chopped (or 2 tablespoons lemon zest + 1 teaspoon salt)
- 3 cloves garlic, minced
- 1/3 cup pistachios, roughly chopped
- 1/4 cup fresh mint, chopped
- 2 tablespoons fresh dill
- 1 tablespoon honey
- Salt and black pepper to taste
- Lemon wedges for serving

DIRECTIONS

1. Preheat oven to 425°F (220°C).
2. Pat salmon dry and season with salt and pepper.
3. Arrange asparagus on large rimmed baking sheet and drizzle with 2 tablespoons olive oil. Season with salt and pepper.
4. In small bowl, combine remaining olive oil, preserved lemons, garlic, pistachios, mint, dill, and honey.
5. Place salmon fillets on baking sheet with asparagus. Top each fillet with herb mixture.
6. Roast 12-15 minutes until salmon flakes easily and asparagus is tender.
7. Serve immediately with lemon wedges.

NUTRITION

Per serving: 195 calories, 3g protein, 24g carbohydrates, 11g fat, 3g fiber

STORAGE

Best served immediately. Leftovers keep for up to 2 days refrigerated.

Thai Curry Chicken with Vegetables

Servings	Prep time	Cook time
6	15 minutes	20 minutes

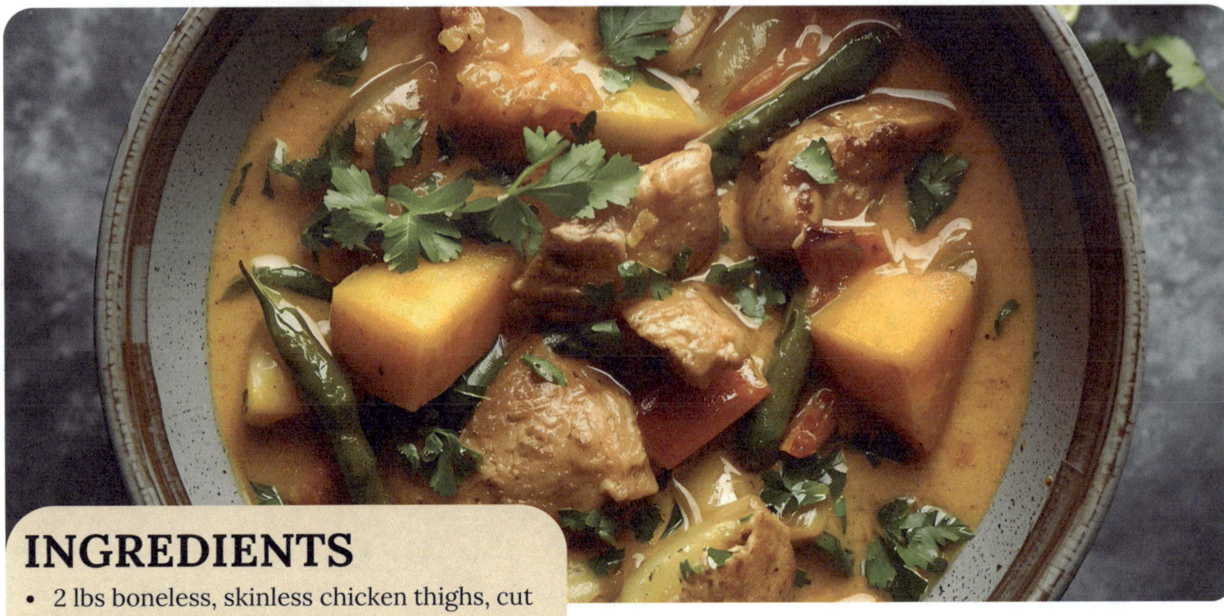

INGREDIENTS

- 2 lbs boneless, skinless chicken thighs, cut into chunks
- 2 tablespoons coconut oil
- 1 medium onion, sliced
- 3 cloves garlic, minced
- 1 tablespoon fresh ginger, minced
- 2-3 tablespoons red curry paste (to taste)
- 1 can (14 oz) coconut milk
- 2 cups butternut squash, cubed
- 1 lb green beans, trimmed and cut into 2-inch pieces
- 1 red bell pepper, sliced
- 2 tablespoons fish sauce
- 1 tablespoon brown sugar
- 2 tablespoons lime juice
- 1/4 cup fresh Thai basil (or regular basil)
- 1/4 cup fresh cilantro
- Lime wedges for serving

NUTRITION

Per serving: 365 calories, 28g protein, 16g carbohydrates, 22g fat, 4g fiber

STORAGE

Keeps for up to 3 days refrigerated. Flavors improve overnight.

Traditional Thai flavors enhanced with unexpected seasonal vegetables that add sweetness and texture to balance the curry heat.

DIRECTIONS

1. Heat coconut oil in large skillet or wok over medium-high heat.
2. Season chicken with salt and pepper. Cook chicken until browned, about 8 minutes. Remove and set aside.
3. Add onion to same pan and cook 4 minutes until softened.
4. Add garlic, ginger, and curry paste. Cook 2 minutes until fragrant.
5. Add coconut milk, scraping up any browned bits.
6. Add butternut squash and bring to simmer. Cook 8 minutes until squash starts to soften.
7. Add green beans, bell pepper, and chicken. Simmer 8-10 minutes until vegetables are tender and chicken is cooked through.
8. Stir in fish sauce, brown sugar, and lime juice.
9. Remove from heat and stir in fresh basil and cilantro.
10. Serve with lime wedges and over cauliflower rice if desired.

Pork Tenderloin with Apples & Fennel

4 | 15 minutes | 25 minutes

Tender pork roasted with sweet apples and aromatic fennel creates an elegant, restaurant-quality meal in one pan.

INGREDIENTS

- 2 pork tenderloins (about 1 1/2 lbs total)
- 2 large fennel bulbs, sliced
- 3 Honeycrisp apples, cored and cut into wedges
- 1 large red onion, sliced
- 1/4 cup olive oil
- 2 tablespoons fresh rosemary, chopped
- 1 tablespoon fresh thyme
- 3 cloves garlic, minced
- 2 tablespoons balsamic vinegar
- 1 tablespoon Dijon mustard
- 1/2 cup white wine (optional)
- Salt and black pepper to taste
- 1/4 cup fresh parsley for garnish

NUTRITION

Per serving: 385 calories, 36g protein, 22g carbohydrates, 18g fat, 6g fiber

STORAGE

Leftovers keep for up to 3 days refrigerated.

DIRECTIONS

1. Preheat oven to 425°F (220°C).
2. Pat pork dry and season generously with salt, pepper, rosemary, and thyme.
3. Heat 2 tablespoons olive oil in large oven-safe skillet over medium-high heat.
4. Sear pork tenderloins on all sides until golden brown, about 8 minutes total. Remove and set aside.
5. Add remaining olive oil to same pan. Add fennel, apples, red onion, and garlic. Cook 5 minutes until starting to soften.
6. In small bowl, whisk together balsamic vinegar, Dijon mustard, and wine (if using).
7. Pour mixture over vegetables and return pork to pan, nestling among vegetables.
8. Transfer to oven and roast 12-15 minutes until pork reaches internal temperature of 145°F (63°C).
9. Let rest 5 minutes before slicing. Garnish with fresh parsley.

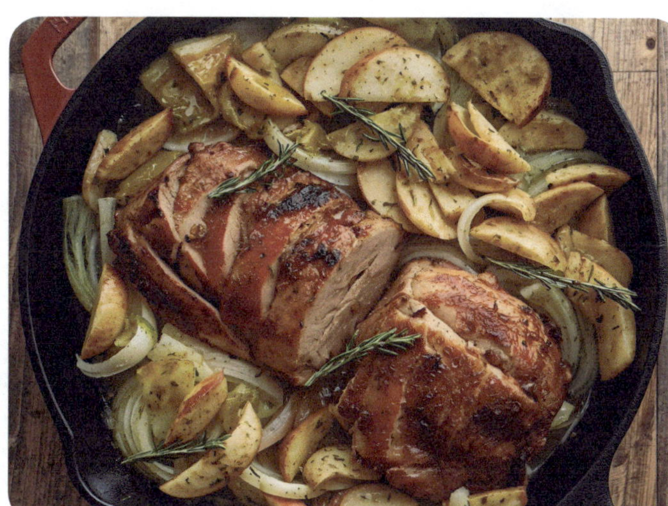

Balsamic Glazed Chicken & Sprouts

6 | 15 minutes | 30 minutes

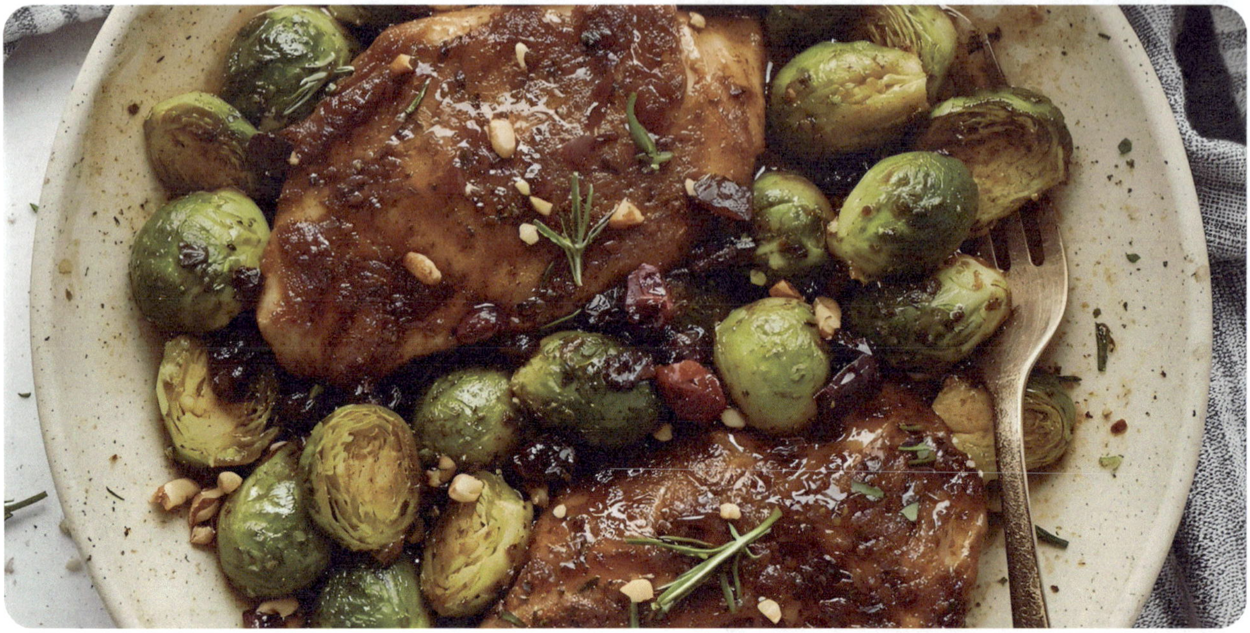

Sweet and tangy balsamic glaze elevates simple chicken and Brussels sprouts into a sophisticated weeknight dinner.

INGREDIENTS

- 6 boneless, skinless chicken breasts
- 1 1/2 lbs Brussels sprouts, halved
- 1/4 cup olive oil
- 1/4 cup balsamic vinegar
- 2 tablespoons honey
- 3 cloves garlic, minced
- 1 tablespoon fresh rosemary, chopped
- 1/2 cup dried cranberries
- 1/3 cup toasted pine nuts
- Salt and black pepper to taste

DIRECTIONS

1. Preheat oven to 425°F (220°C).
2. Season chicken breasts with salt and pepper.
3. Heat 2 tablespoons olive oil in large oven-safe skillet over medium-high heat.
4. Sear chicken breasts 3-4 minutes per side until golden. Remove and set aside.
5. Add Brussels sprouts to same pan with remaining olive oil. Season with salt and pepper.
6. In small bowl, whisk together balsamic vinegar, honey, garlic, and rosemary.
7. Return chicken to pan, nestling among Brussels sprouts.
8. Pour balsamic mixture over chicken and vegetables.
9. Transfer to oven and roast 18-20 minutes until chicken reaches 165°F (74°C) and Brussels sprouts are tender.
10. Sprinkle with cranberries and pine nuts during last 5 minutes of cooking.

NUTRITION

Per serving: 365 calories, 35g protein, 18g carbohydrates, 17g fat, 5g fiber

STORAGE

Leftovers keep for up to 3 days refrigerated.

Moroccan-Spiced Cod with Vegetables

Flaky white fish seasoned with warm Moroccan spices and roasted with colorful vegetables creates an exotic yet accessible dinner.

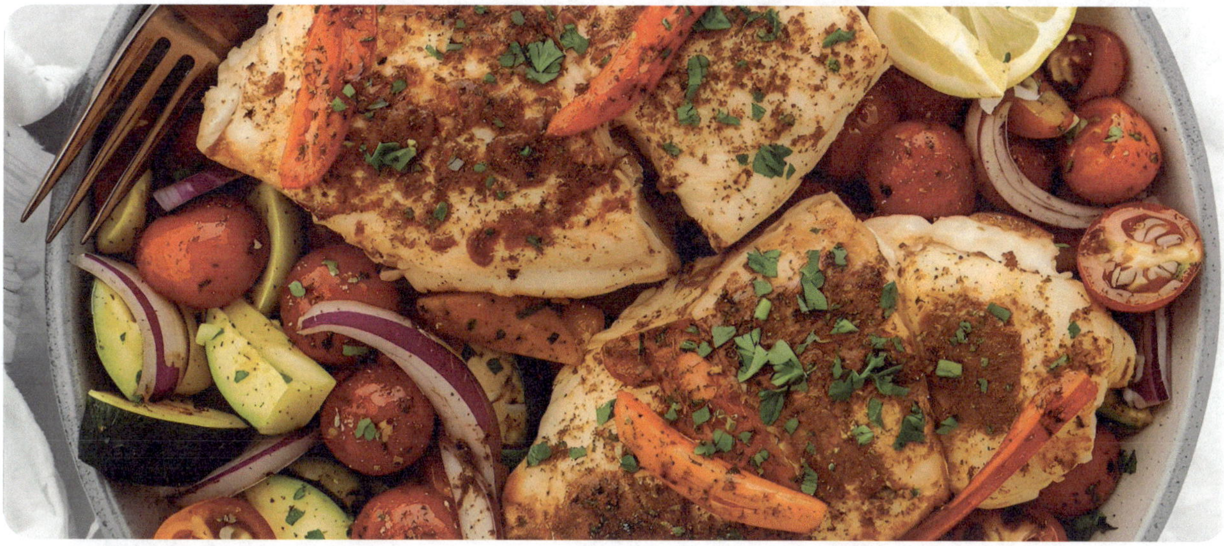

INGREDIENTS

- 4 cod fillets (6 oz each)
- 2 bell peppers (different colors), sliced
- 1 large zucchini, sliced
- 1 red onion, sliced
- 1 pint cherry tomatoes
- 1/4 cup olive oil
- 2 teaspoons ground coriander
- 1 teaspoon ground cumin
- 1 teaspoon paprika
- 1/2 teaspoon cinnamon
- 1/2 teaspoon ground ginger
- 1/4 teaspoon cayenne pepper
- 3 cloves garlic, minced
- 1/4 cup fresh cilantro, chopped
- 2 tablespoons lemon juice
- Salt and black pepper to taste
- Lemon wedges for serving

4 | 15 minutes | 20 minutes

DIRECTIONS

1. Preheat oven to 425°F (220°C).
2. In small bowl, combine coriander, cumin, paprika, cinnamon, ginger, cayenne, salt, and pepper.
3. Pat cod fillets dry and rub with half the spice mixture.
4. Toss vegetables with olive oil, garlic, and remaining spice mixture.
5. Arrange vegetables on large rimmed baking sheet and roast 10 minutes.
6. Add cod fillets to baking sheet and continue roasting 8-10 minutes until fish flakes easily.
7. Drizzle with lemon juice and sprinkle with cilantro.
8. Serve with lemon wedges.

NUTRITION

Per serving: 285 calories, 32g protein, 12g carbohydrates, 12g fat, 4g fiber

STORAGE

Best served immediately. Leftovers keep for up to 2 days refrigerated.

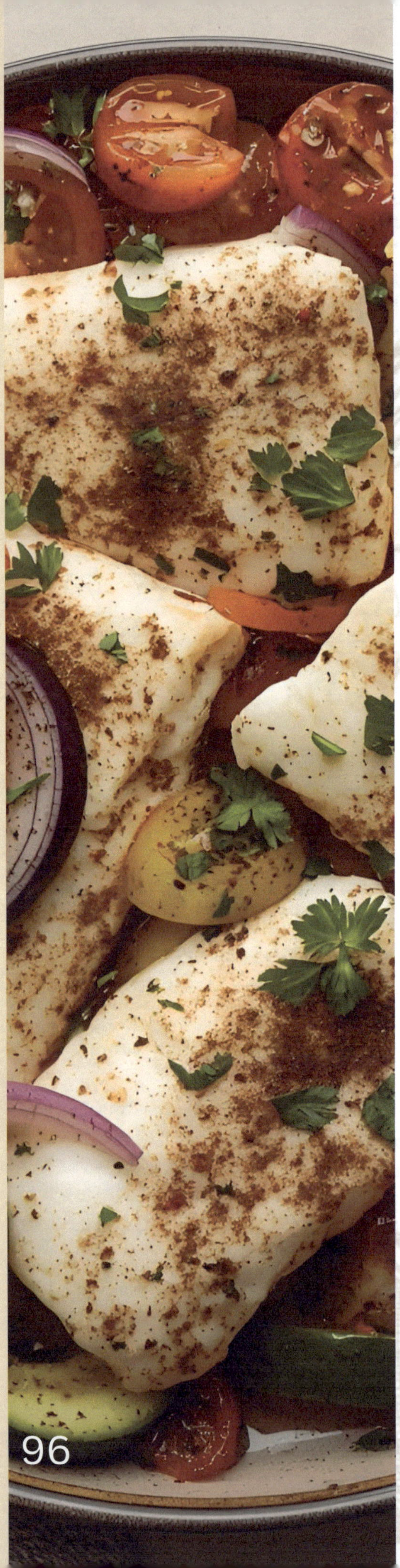

TIPS FOR ONE-PAN SUCCESS

Timing is Everything: Add ingredients in order of cooking time required. Dense vegetables need more time than delicate fish or quick-cooking greens.

Don't Overcrowd: Use large enough pans to allow proper browning and even cooking. Multiple smaller pans are better than one overcrowded pan.

Temperature Control: Start with high heat for browning, then adjust as needed. Most one-pan meals benefit from initial searing followed by gentler cooking.

Layer Flavors: Season at multiple stages and use fond (browned bits) to build depth. Deglaze with wine, broth, or citrus juice to capture all the flavor.

Prepare Mise en Place: Have all ingredients prepped before you start cooking. One-pan meals move quickly once you begin.

Choose the Right Pan: Heavy-bottomed, oven-safe skillets or Dutch ovens work best. Cast iron retains heat beautifully for searing and roasting.

Rest When Needed: Allow proteins to rest after cooking for optimal texture and juice retention.

Finish with Fresh Elements: Add fresh herbs, citrus juice, or quality olive oil at the end to brighten flavors and add visual appeal.

Scale Appropriately: These recipes can usually be halved or doubled successfully. Adjust pan size and cooking times accordingly.

Embrace Leftovers: Most one-pan meals reheat well and often develop even better flavors overnight. Perfect for meal prep and easy lunches.

One-pan cooking is as much about technique as it is about convenience. Master these principles and you'll be able to create satisfying, complete meals with minimal effort and maximum flavor.

CHAPTER 09

Slow & Pressure Cooker Meals

The magic of hands-off cooking lies in transforming tough cuts of meat into fork-tender centerpieces while building complex flavors through time and gentle heat. Whether you prefer the leisurely approach of slow cooking or the speed of pressure cooking, these appliances excel at creating deeply satisfying meals with minimal active cooking time. Each recipe provides instructions for both methods, allowing you to choose based on your schedule and preferences. The key to success lies in understanding how ingredients behave under pressure or extended cooking, layering flavors appropriately, and finishing dishes with fresh elements that brighten and complete each meal.

List of Recipes

Chicken and White Bean Chili

Tender beef with a sweet-savory glaze that caramelizes beautifully on the grill.

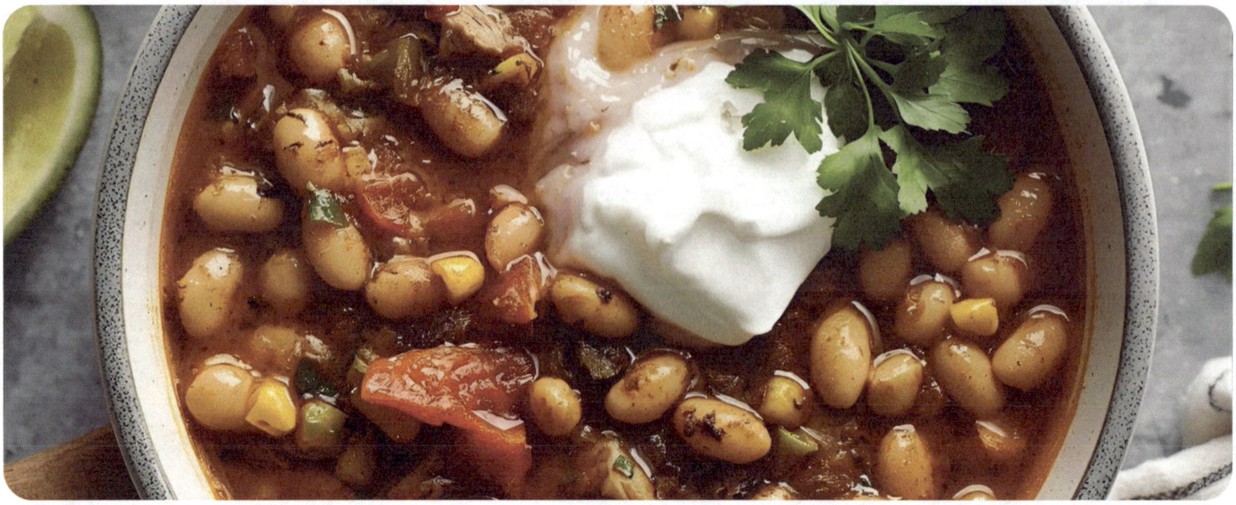

INGREDIENTS

- 2 lbs boneless, skinless chicken thighs
- 3 cans (15 oz each) white beans, drained and rinsed
- 1 large onion, diced
- 2 bell peppers, diced
- 4 cloves garlic, minced
- 2 cans (4 oz each) diced green chiles
- 3 cups chicken broth
- 2 teaspoons ground cumin
- 1 teaspoon chili powder
- 1 teaspoon oregano
- 1/2 teaspoon smoked paprika
- 1/4 teaspoon cayenne pepper
- 1 cup frozen corn
- 1/4 cup fresh cilantro, chopped
- 2 tablespoons lime juice
- Salt and black pepper to taste
- Avocado, Greek yogurt, and lime wedges for serving

8	15 minutes	4-6 hour on low	15 minutes

DIRECTIONS

Slow Cooker Method:

1. Place chicken thighs in slow cooker and season with salt and pepper.
2. Add onion, bell peppers, garlic, green chiles, white beans, and broth.
3. Stir in cumin, chili powder, oregano, paprika, and cayenne.
4. Cook on low 4-6 hours until chicken is tender and easily shreds.
5. Remove chicken, shred with forks, and return to pot.
6. Add corn and cook 15 minutes more.
7. Stir in cilantro and lime juice before serving.

Pressure Cooker Method:

1. Add all ingredients except corn, cilantro, and lime juice to pressure cooker.
2. Pressure cook on high 15 minutes, quick release.
3. Remove chicken, shred, and return to pot.
4. Add corn and simmer on sauté function for 5 minutes.
5. Stir in cilantro and lime juice.

NUTRITION

Per serving: 295 calories, 28g protein, 32g carbohydrates, 6g fat, 8g fiber

STORAGE

Freezes for up to 3 months without dairy toppings.

Moroccan Lamb Tagine

Exotic spices and unexpected pomegranate sweetness create a sophisticated dish that transports you to North African markets.

Servings	Prep time	Slow cooker	Pressure cooker
5	20 minutes	6-7 hours on low	35 minutes

NUTRITION

Per serving: 425 calories, 35g protein, 18g carbohydrates, 24g fat, 4g fiber

STORAGE

Improves with time. Keeps for up to 4 days refrigerated.

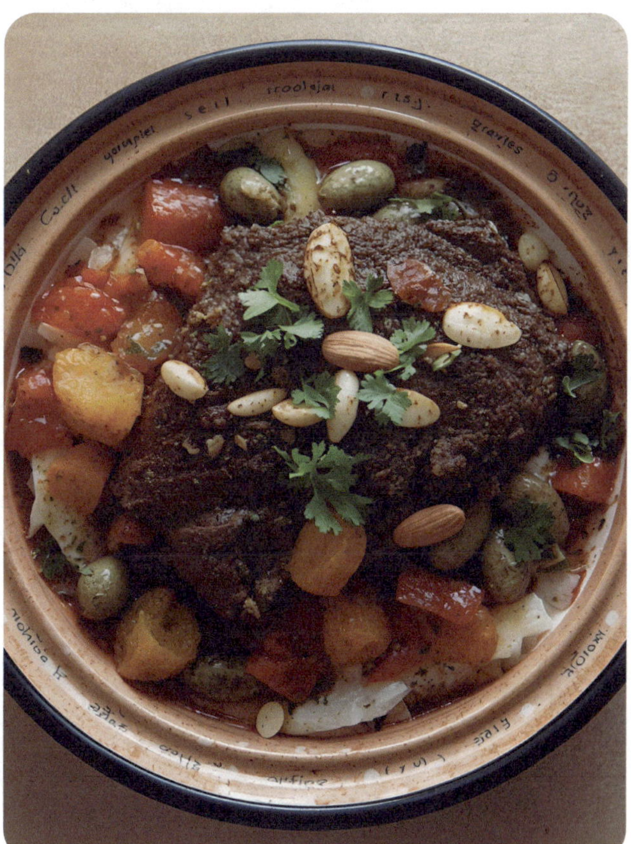

INGREDIENTS

- 3 lbs lamb shoulder, cut into chunks
- 2 large onions, sliced
- 4 cloves garlic, minced
- 1 tablespoon fresh ginger, minced
- 2 teaspoons ground cinnamon
- 2 teaspoons ground ginger
- 1 teaspoon turmeric
- 1 teaspoon ground coriander
- 1/2 teaspoon ground cumin
- 1/4 teaspoon cayenne pepper
- 1 can (14 oz) diced tomatoes
- 1 cup low sodium chicken broth
- 2 tablespoons pomegranate molasses
- 1/2 cup dried apricots, chopped
- 1/2 cup pitted green olives
- 1/3 cup sliced almonds, toasted
- 1/4 cup fresh mint, chopped
- 1/4 cup fresh cilantro, chopped
- Salt and black pepper to taste

DIRECTIONS

Slow Cooker Method:

1. Season lamb chunks with salt and pepper.
2. In large skillet, brown lamb in batches over medium-high heat, about 8 minutes total. Transfer to slow cooker.
3. Add onions to same skillet and cook until softened, about 6 minutes. Add garlic and fresh ginger, cooking 1 minute more.
4. Add all spices and cook until fragrant, about 1 minute. Transfer to slow cooker.
5. Add tomatoes, broth, pomegranate molasses, and apricots to slow cooker.
6. Cook on low 6-7 hours until lamb is tender.
7. Add olives during last 30 minutes of cooking.

Garnish with toasted almonds, mint, and cilantro before serving.

Pressure Cooker Method:

1. Brown lamb using sauté function, then set aside.
2. Sauté onions, garlic, ginger, and spices as above.
3. Return lamb to pot with remaining ingredients except olives and garnishes.
4. Pressure cook on high 35 minutes, natural release 15 minutes.
5. Stir in olives and garnish before serving.

Pork Shoulder with Apples and Sauerkraut

8	15 minutes	8 hours on low	15 minutes

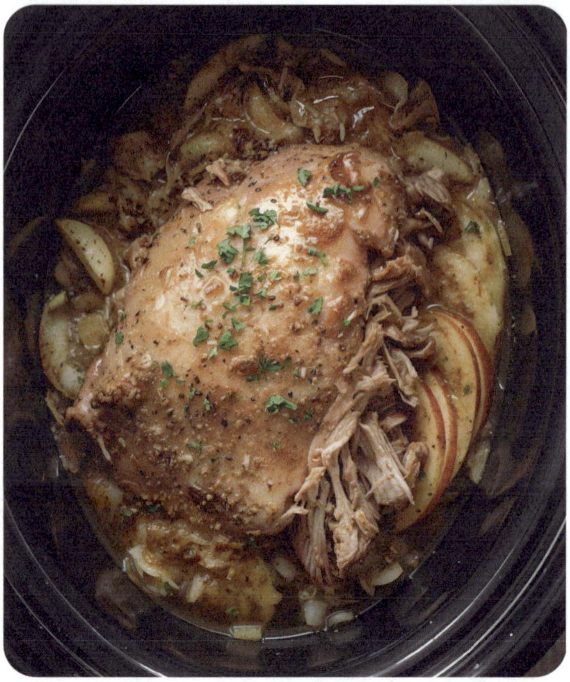

German-inspired comfort food with tender pork, tangy sauerkraut, and sweet apples creating perfect flavor balance.

INGREDIENTS

- 4 lb pork shoulder, trimmed
- 2 lbs sauerkraut, drained
- 3 large apples, cored and sliced
- 1 large onion, sliced
- 3 cloves garlic, minced
- 2 cups chicken broth
- 1/4 cup apple cider vinegar
- 2 tablespoons brown mustard
- 2 teaspoons caraway seeds
- 1 teaspoon smoked paprika
- 2 bay leaves
- Salt and black pepper to taste
- Fresh parsley for garnish

DIRECTIONS

Slow Cooker Method:

1. Season pork shoulder generously with salt and pepper.
2. Layer sauerkraut, apples, and onion in slow cooker.
3. In bowl, whisk together broth, vinegar, mustard, garlic, caraway seeds, and paprika.
4. Place pork on top of vegetables and pour broth mixture over.
5. Add bay leaves and cook on low 8 hours until pork shreds easily.
6. Remove pork, shred with forks, and return to pot.
7. To serve, remove bay leaves and garnish with parsley.

Pressure Cooker Method:

1. Season pork and place in pressure cooker.
2. Add all remaining ingredients except parsley.
3. Pressure cook on high 90 minutes, natural release 20 minutes.
4. Shred pork and mix with cooking juices.
5. To serve, remove bay leaves and garnish with parsley.

NUTRITION
Per serving: 365 calories, 35g protein, 12g carbohydrates, 19g fat, 4g fiber

STORAGE
Keeps for up to 4 days refrigerated or 3 months frozen.

6	15 minutes plus 2 hours chilling	4-5 hours on low	15 minutes

Turkey and Vegetable Curry

Warming Indian spices combined with unexpected vegetables and a bright coconut-lime finish create a unique curry experience.

INGREDIENTS

- 2 lbs turkey thighs, boneless and skinless, cut into chunks
- 2 cups butternut squash, peeled and cubed
- 1 lb green beans, trimmed and cut into 2-inch pieces
- 1 large onion, diced
- 4 cloves garlic, minced
- 1 tablespoon fresh ginger, minced
- 2 tablespoons curry powder
- 1 teaspoon ground coriander
- 1/2 teaspoon turmeric
- 1/4 teaspoon cayenne pepper
- 1 can (14 oz) coconut milk
- 1 can (14 oz) diced tomatoes
- 1 cup chicken broth
- 2 tablespoons tomato paste
- 2 tablespoons lime juice
- 1/4 cup fresh cilantro, chopped
- Salt and black pepper to taste

NUTRITION

Per serving: 325 calories, 30g protein, 16g carbohydrates, 16g fat, 5g fiber

STORAGE

Keeps for up to 3 days refrigerated. Add fresh herbs when reheating.

DIRECTIONS

Slow Cooker Method:

1. Season turkey chunks with salt and pepper.
2. Add turkey, butternut squash, onion, garlic, and ginger to slow cooker.
3. Stir in curry powder, coriander, turmeric, and cayenne.
4. Add coconut milk, diced tomatoes, broth, and tomato paste.
5. Cook on low 4-5 hours until turkey is tender.
6. Add green beans during last 45 minutes of cooking.
7. Stir in lime juice and cilantro before serving.

Pressure Cooker Method:

1. Add all ingredients except green beans, lime juice, and cilantro to pressure cooker.
2. Pressure cook on high 15 minutes, quick release.
3. Add green beans and simmer on sauté function 8-10 minutes until tender.
4. Stir in lime juice and cilantro.

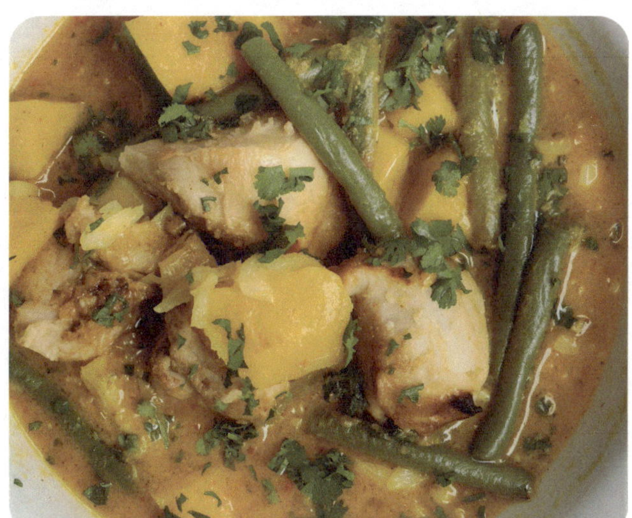

Italian Beef with Peppers

Tender, flavorful beef perfect for serving over zucchini noodles or in lettuce cups for a satisfying, low-carb meal.

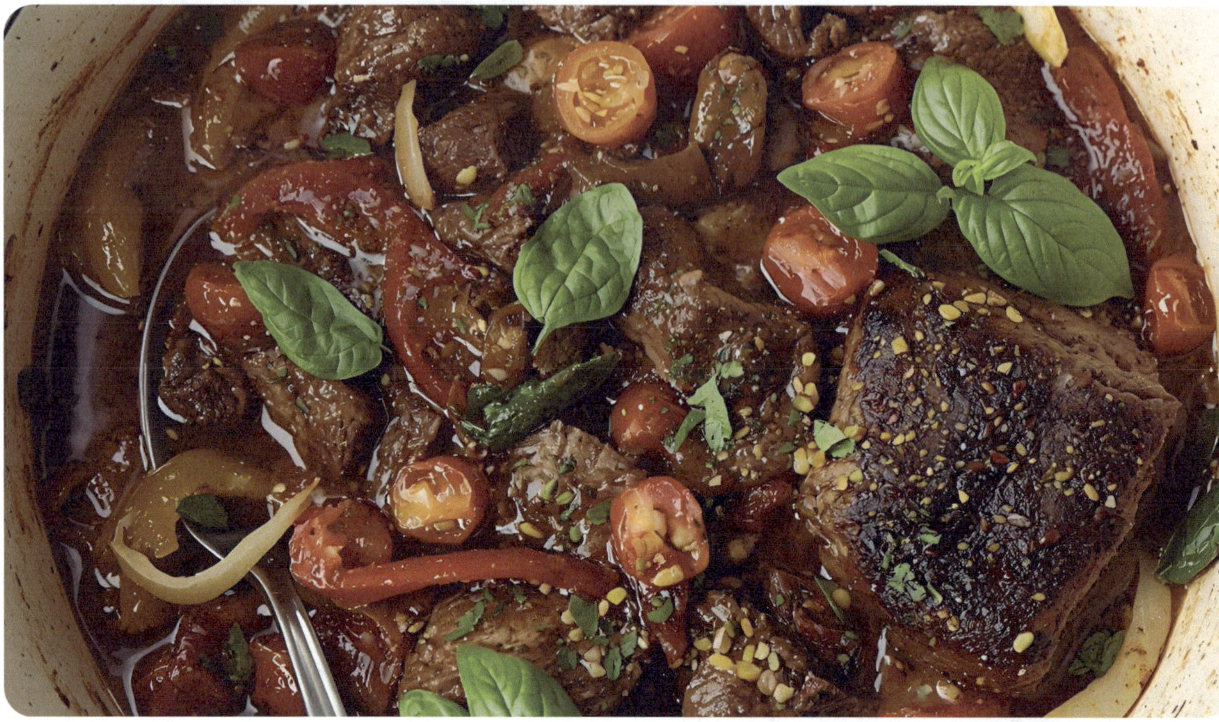

Servings	Prep time	Slow cooker	Pressure cooker
8	15 minutes	8 hours on low	45 minutes

INGREDIENTS

- 4 lb beef chuck roast
- 3 bell peppers (mixed colors), sliced
- 1 large onion, sliced
- 6 cloves garlic, minced
- 1 can (14 oz) diced tomatoes
- 1/2 cup beef broth
- 1/4 cup red wine vinegar
- 2 tablespoons Italian seasoning
- 1 tablespoon oregano
- 2 teaspoons garlic powder
- 1 teaspoon red pepper flakes
- 2 bay leaves
- Salt and black pepper to taste
- Fresh basil for garnish

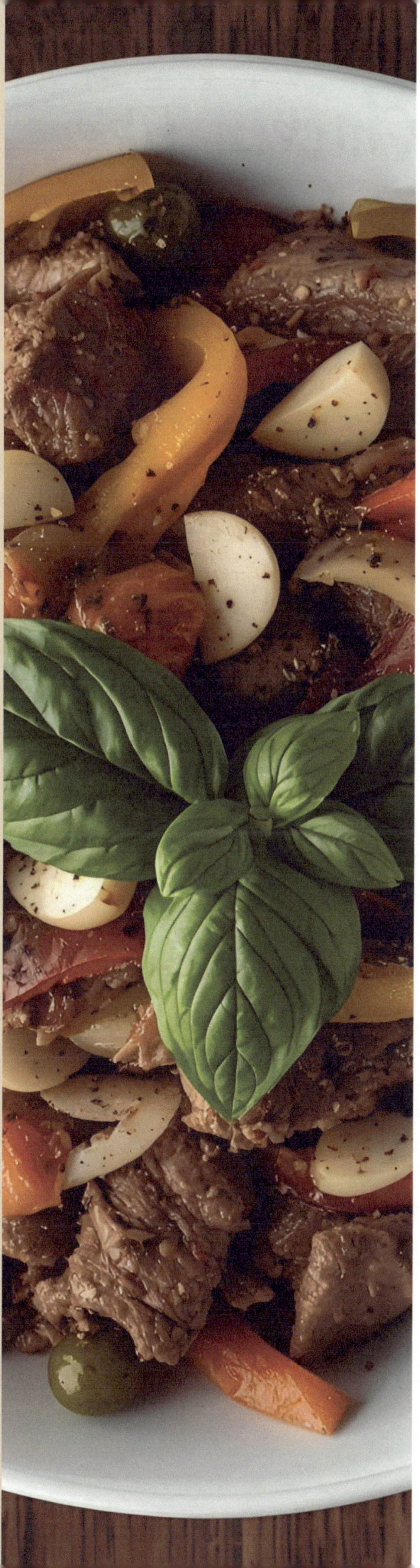

DIRECTION

Slow Cooker Method:

1. Season beef roast generously with salt and pepper.
2. Place beef in slow cooker and surround with bell peppers and onion.
3. In bowl, combine garlic, diced tomatoes, broth, vinegar, Italian seasoning, oregano, garlic powder, and red pepper flakes.
4. Pour mixture over beef and vegetables. Add bay leaves.
5. Cook on low 8 hours until beef shreds easily.
6. Remove beef, shred with forks, and return to pot.
7. To serve, remove bay leaves and garnish with fresh basil.

Pressure Cooker Method:

1. Season beef and place in pressure cooker with vegetables.
2. Add remaining ingredients except basil.
3. Pressure cook on high 45 minutes, natural release 20 minutes.
4. Shred beef and mix with cooking juices.
5. To serve, remove bay leaves and garnish with basil.

NUTRITION

Per serving: 345 calories, 35g protein, 8g carbohydrates, 18g fat, 2g fiber

STORAGE

Freezes beautifully for up to 4 months.

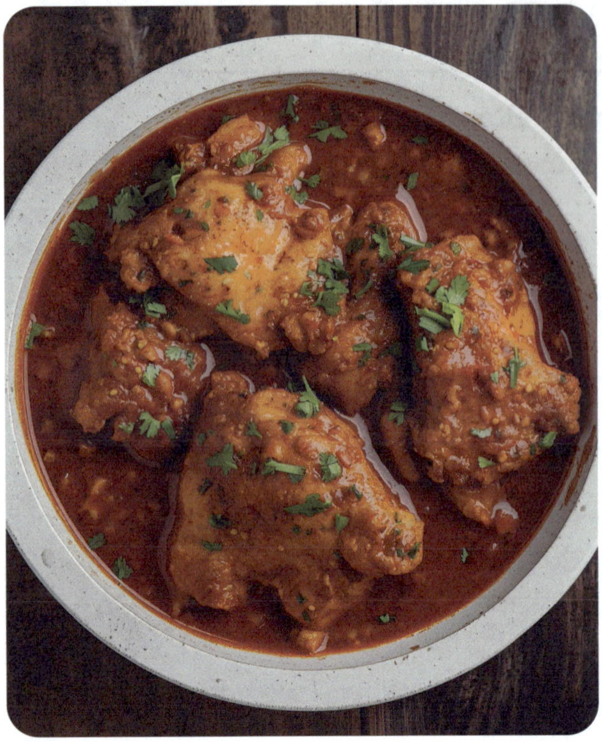

Chicken Tikka Masala

Servings	Prep time	Slow cooker	Pressure cooker
6	25 minutes	4-5 hours on low	12 minutes

Rich, creamy Indian curry with tender chicken in an aromatic tomato-based sauce.

NUTRITION

Per serving: 385 calories, 32g protein, 14g carbohydrates, 22g fat, 3g fiber

STORAGE

Keeps for up to 4 days refrigerated. Flavors improve overnight.

INGREDIENTS

- 3 lbs boneless, skinless chicken thighs, cut into chunks
- 1 large onion, diced
- 4 cloves garlic, minced
- 1 tablespoon fresh ginger, minced
- 2 tablespoons garam masala
- 1 tablespoon ground cumin
- 1 teaspoon turmeric
- 1 teaspoon smoked paprika
- 1/2 teaspoon cayenne pepper
- 1 can (28 oz) crushed tomatoes
- 1 can (14 oz) coconut milk
- 2 tablespoons tomato paste
- 1 tablespoon brown sugar
- 1/2 cup heavy cream
- 1/4 cup fresh cilantro, chopped
- Salt and black pepper to taste

DIRECTIONS

Slow Cooker Method:

1. Season chicken chunks with salt and pepper.
2. In large skillet, brown chicken in batches over medium-high heat, about 6 minutes total. Transfer to slow cooker.
3. Add onion to same skillet and cook until softened. Add garlic, ginger, and all spices, cooking 2 minutes until fragrant.
4. Add crushed tomatoes, coconut milk, tomato paste, and brown sugar. Transfer to slow cooker.
5. Cook on low 4-5 hours until chicken is tender.
6. Stir in heavy cream during last 30 minutes.
7. Garnish with cilantro before serving.

Pressure Cooker Method:

1. Brown chicken using sauté function, then set aside.
2. Sauté onion, garlic, ginger, and spices as above.
3. Return chicken to pot with remaining ingredients except cream and cilantro.
4. Pressure cook on high 12 minutes, quick release.
5. Stir in cream and garnish with cilantro.

Mediterranean Fish Stew

Servings	Prep time	Cook time
6	20 minutes	2-3 hours on low

Light, flavorful stew with tender fish and vegetables in a tomato-herb broth.

INGREDIENTS

- 2 lbs firm white fish (halibut, cod), cut into chunks
- 1 large onion, diced
- 1 bell pepper, diced
- 4 cloves garlic, minced
- 1 can (28 oz) diced tomatoes
- 2 cups fish stock or chicken broth
- 1/2 cup white wine (optional)
- 2 tablespoons tomato paste
- 2 teaspoons dried oregano
- 1 teaspoon dried thyme
- 1/2 teaspoon red pepper flakes
- 1/2 cup Kalamata olives, pitted
- 1/4 cup capers
- 1/4 cup fresh parsley, chopped
- 2 tablespoons fresh dill
- Salt and black pepper to taste
- Lemon wedges for serving

DIRECTIONS

Slow Cooker Method:

1. Add onion, bell pepper, garlic, diced tomatoes, stock, wine, tomato paste, oregano, thyme, and red pepper flakes to slow cooker.
2. Cook on low 2-3 hours until vegetables are tender.
3. Season fish chunks with salt and pepper.
4. Add fish, olives, and capers to slow cooker.
5. Cook 30-45 minutes more until fish flakes easily.
6. Stir in fresh herbs and serve with lemon wedges.

Pressure Cooker Method:

1. Add vegetables, tomatoes, stock, wine, and seasonings to pressure cooker.
2. Pressure cook on high 5 minutes, quick release.
3. Add fish, olives, and capers.
4. Simmer on sauté function 8-10 minutes until fish is cooked.
5. Stir in herbs and serve with lemon.

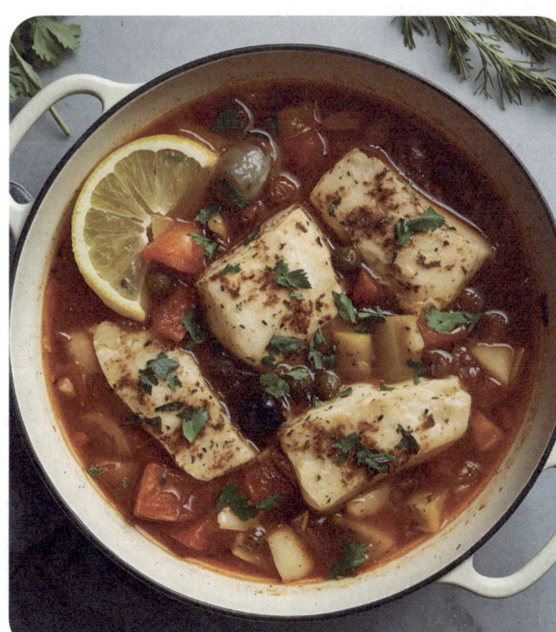

NUTRITION

Per serving: 245 calories, 32g protein, 12g carbohydrates, 6g fat, 3g fiber

STORAGE

Best consumed within 2 days. Fish texture may change with longer storage.

Asian-Style Short Ribs

Warming Indian spices combined with unexpected vegetables and a bright coconut-lime finish create a unique curry experience.

6	15 minutes	8 hours on low	45 minutes

INGREDIENTS

- 4 lbs beef short ribs, cut into individual ribs
- 1/4 cup low-sodium soy sauce (gluten-free)
- 1/4 cup rice vinegar
- 2 tablespoons honey
- 2 tablespoons sesame oil
- 1 tablespoon fresh ginger, minced
- 4 cloves garlic, minced
- 1 onion, sliced
- 2 star anise pods
- 1 cinnamon stick
- 1/4 teaspoon red pepper flakes
- 2 green onions, sliced
- 1 tablespoon sesame seeds
- Fresh cilantro for garnish

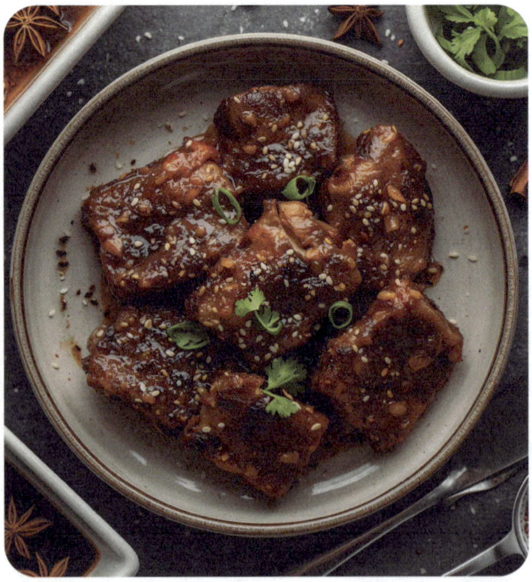

DIRECTIONS

Slow Cooker Method:

1. Season short ribs with salt and pepper.
2. In large skillet, brown ribs on all sides over medium-high heat, about 10 minutes total. Transfer to slow cooker.
3. In bowl, whisk together soy sauce, rice vinegar, honey, sesame oil, ginger, and garlic.
4. Add onion, star anise, cinnamon stick, and red pepper flakes to slow cooker.
5. Pour sauce mixture over ribs.
6. Cook on low 8 hours until meat falls off the bone.
7. Remove whole spices and garnish with green onions, sesame seeds, and cilantro.

Pressure Cooker Method:

1. Brown ribs using sauté function, then set aside.
2. Add sauce ingredients and aromatics to pot.
3. Return ribs to pot and pressure cook on high 45 minutes, natural release 15 minutes.
4. Remove spices and garnish as above.

NUTRITION

Per serving: 485 calories, 42g protein, 8g carbohydrates, 32g fat, 1g fiber

STORAGE

Keeps for up to 4 days refrigerated. Remove from bone before storing.

Vegetarian Lentil Stew

Hearty, protein-rich stew packed with vegetables and warming spices that satisfies meat-eaters and vegetarians alike.

Servings	Prep time	Cook time	Pressure cooker
8	20 minutes	6-7 hours on low	15 minutes

INGREDIENTS

- 2 cups dried green lentils, rinsed
- 2 large carrots, diced
- 2 celery stalks, diced
- 1 large onion, diced
- 1 bell pepper, diced
- 4 cloves garlic, minced
- 1 can (28 oz) diced tomatoes
- 4 cups vegetable broth
- 2 bay leaves
- 2 teaspoons ground cumin
- 1 teaspoon smoked paprika
- 1 teaspoon dried thyme
- 1/2 teaspoon turmeric
- 2 cups fresh spinach, chopped
- 1/4 cup fresh parsley, chopped
- 2 tablespoons lemon juice
- Salt and black pepper to taste

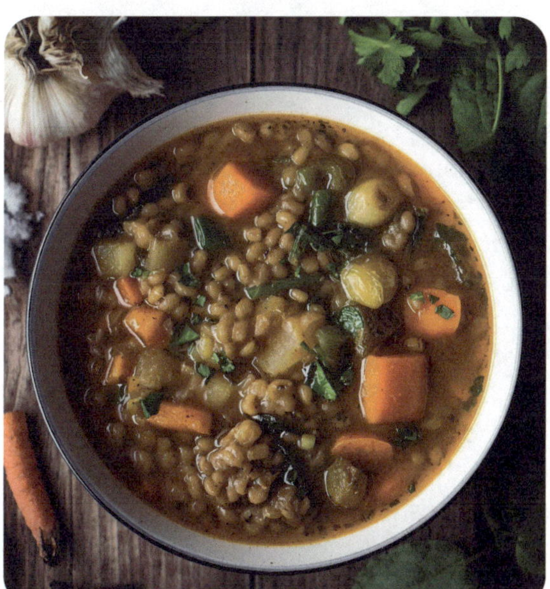

DIRECTIONS

Slow Cooker Method:

1. Add lentils, carrots, celery, onion, bell pepper, and garlic to slow cooker.
2. Stir in diced tomatoes, broth, bay leaves, cumin, paprika, thyme, and turmeric.
3. Cook on low 6-7 hours until lentils are tender.
4. Add spinach during last 15 minutes of cooking.
5. Remove bay leaves and stir in parsley and lemon juice.
6. Season with salt and pepper to taste.

Pressure Cooker Method:

1. Add all ingredients except spinach, parsley, and lemon juice to pressure cooker.
2. Pressure cook on high 15 minutes, natural release 10 minutes.
3. Stir in spinach until wilted.
4. Add parsley and lemon juice, then season to taste.

NUTRITION

Per serving: 215 calories, 14g protein, 38g carbohydrates, 2g fat, 9g fiber

STORAGE

Freezes beautifully for up to 4 months. Add fresh herbs when reheating

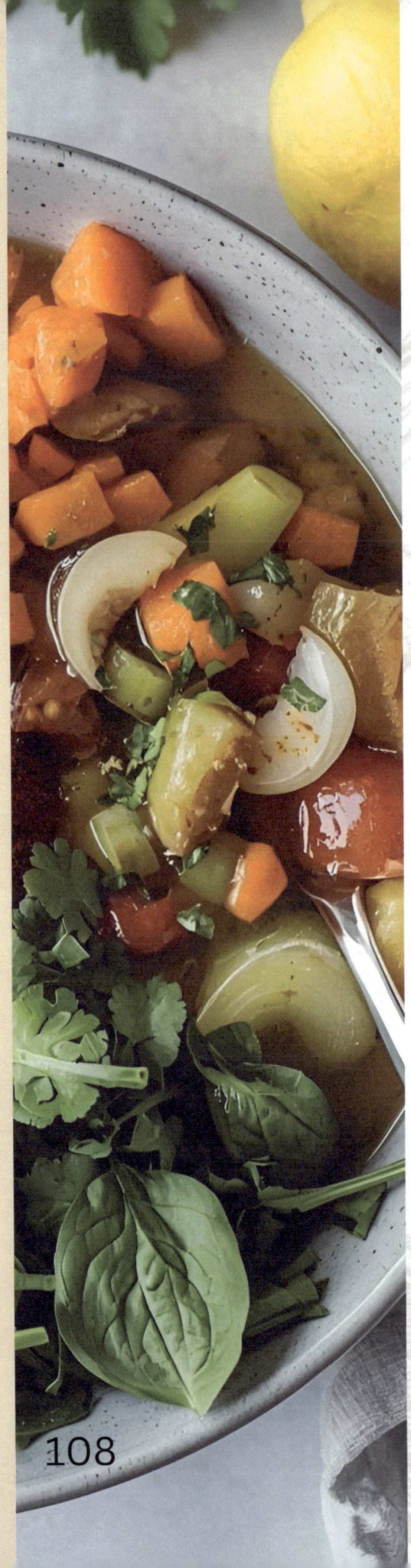

TIPS FOR SLOW AND PRESSURE COOKER SUCCESS

Layer Flavors Properly: Brown meats and sauté aromatics when possible before adding to the cooker. This builds foundational flavors that can't be achieved through long cooking alone.

Liquid Ratios: Slow cookers need less liquid than stovetop cooking since little evaporates. Pressure cookers need minimum liquid amounts for proper function – usually 1-2 cups depending on size.

Timing Adjustments: Dense vegetables like potatoes and carrots take longer to cook than proteins. Add delicate vegetables like spinach or peas during the last portion of cooking time.

Natural vs. Quick Release: Tough cuts of meat benefit from natural pressure release, which continues gentle cooking. Quick release works well for vegetables and fish.

Finish with Fresh Elements: Both methods benefit from finishing touches – fresh herbs, citrus juice, or quality olive oil added after cooking brightens flavors.

Size Matters: Don't overfill cookers – maximum 2/3 full for slow cookers, 1/2 to 2/3 for pressure cookers to allow proper circulation.

Dairy Additions: Add cream, yogurt, or cheese during the last 30 minutes of slow cooking or after pressure cooking to prevent curdling.

Thickening Strategies: Use almond flour, pureed vegetables, or tomato paste rather than wheat flour for gluten-free thickening.

Meal Prep Advantages: Both methods excel at batch cooking. Make large batches and freeze in family-sized portions for easy future meals.

Convert Traditional Recipes: Reduce liquid by 1/3 for slow cooker conversions, reduce cooking time dramatically for pressure cooker versions (roughly 1/3 of original time under pressure).

Both of these cooking methods have a forgiving nature and excel at transforming inexpensive ingredients into restaurant-quality meals with minimal hands-on time.

CHAPTER 10
Reinventing Rice

List of Recipes

1. Cajun Cauliflower Jambalaya
2. Parmesan Mushroom Risotto
3. Shrimp and Edamame Fried Rice
4. Cheesy Chicken and Broccoli Skillet
5. Smokey Mexican Beef and Cauliflower Rice
6. Tex-Mex Cauliflower & Black Bean Bowl
7. Lemon-Herb Cauliflower & Quinoa Pilaf
8. Coconut Curry Shrimp with Green Beans
9. Pesto Shrimp "Pasotto"

Rice was always one of my kitchen mainstays—flexible, comforting, and the perfect base for so many of my favorite dishes. When my doctor suggested cutting back to help manage my blood sugar, I'll admit, I was skeptical. How could I give up something so central to my meals? But necessity, as they say, is the mother of invention. Over time, I discovered that vegetable rices—especially cauliflower rice—were not just a passable stand-in, but an upgrade in many ways. They cook up in a fraction of the time, absorb flavors beautifully, and, truthfully, I rarely find myself missing the real thing.

I quickly learned that cauliflower is just the beginning. There's a whole world of low-carb, blood sugar-friendly alternatives out there! Broccoli rice adds a vibrant color and a nutritional powerhouse punch (hello, extra fiber and folate!). Hearts of palm rice brings a delicate, slightly nutty flavor and a texture somewhere between rice and pasta—perfect for salads or creamy dishes. Konjac rice (sometimes labeled shirataki rice) is a game-changer for those looking for the lowest carb option; it's mild in taste, but soaks up sauces beautifully and gives you the chewy satisfaction of rice without any blood sugar worries.

One of the unexpected joys of this swap is how forgiving these vegetable rices can be. Unlike grain rice, which can go from perfect to sticky or mushy in a blink, cauliflower and its cousins seem to shrug off my occasional distracted cooking. They're just as happy in a skillet as in a casserole, and it's surprisingly hard to overcook them. I love that I can make a big batch from scratch if I'm feeling ambitious, or keep my freezer and pantry stocked with pre-riced vegetables (and even ready-to-use konjac!) for those nights when time is short. There's no shame in the convenience game—both options help me stay on track without feeling deprived.

This chapter is packed with some of my favorite ways to turn cauliflower and other veggie rices into satisfying main courses that never feel like "diet food." I've taken inspiration from comfort classics and global favorites, finding that these new bases make old flavors shine in fresh, healthy ways. Whether you're cooking for one or feeding a crowd, I hope these recipes help you rediscover the joy of a hearty bowl—without the blood sugar worries. Trust me, with a little creativity and an open mind to the variety of rice substitutes out there, you might just find yourself a fan of the swap too.

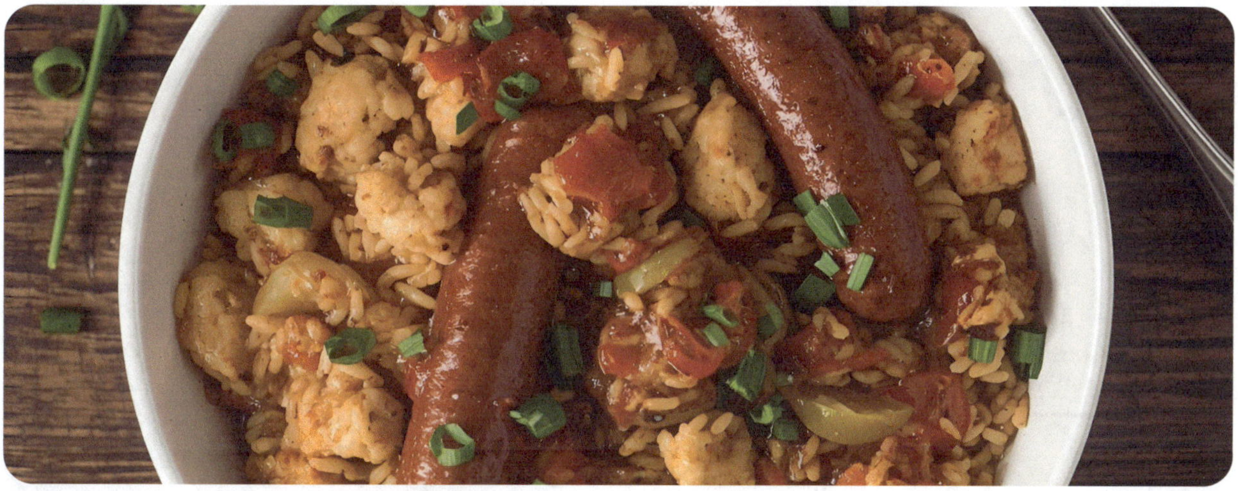

Cajun Cauliflower Jambalaya

6	20 minutes	35 minutes

INGREDIENTS

- 1 large cauliflower, riced (about 5 cups)
- 12 oz andouille sausage, sliced
- 2 boneless, skinless chicken thighs, diced
- 1 onion, diced
- 1 bell pepper, diced
- 2 stalks celery, diced
- 3 cloves garlic, minced
- 1 can (14.5 oz) diced tomatoes, undrained
- 2 cups gluten-free chicken broth
- 2 tbsp Cajun seasoning
- 1 tsp smoked paprika
- Salt and pepper
- Hot sauce to taste
- Chopped scallions and parsley for garnish

Enjoy the bold tastes of Louisiana with hearty jambalaya, made with rice, smoky sausage, tender chicken, and vibrant peppers for a flavorful kick.

DIRECTIONS

1. In a large skillet or Dutch oven, brown sausage and chicken over medium-high heat; remove and set aside.
2. In the same pan, sauté onion, bell pepper, celery, and garlic until softened, about 8 minutes.
3. Stir in cauliflower rice, tomatoes, broth, Cajun seasoning, smoked paprika, salt, and pepper.
4. Bring to a simmer, then add sausage and chicken back to the pan.
5. Cook, uncovered, 20–25 min until cauliflower is tender and liquid is absorbed.
6. Adjust seasoning and stir in hot sauce to taste.
7. Garnish with scallions and parsley.

NUTRITION

Per serving: 340 calories, 24g protein, 18g carbohydrates, 18g fat, 6g fiber

STORAGE

Keeps refrigerated for up to 4 days or frozen for 3 months.

Parmesan Mushroom Risotto

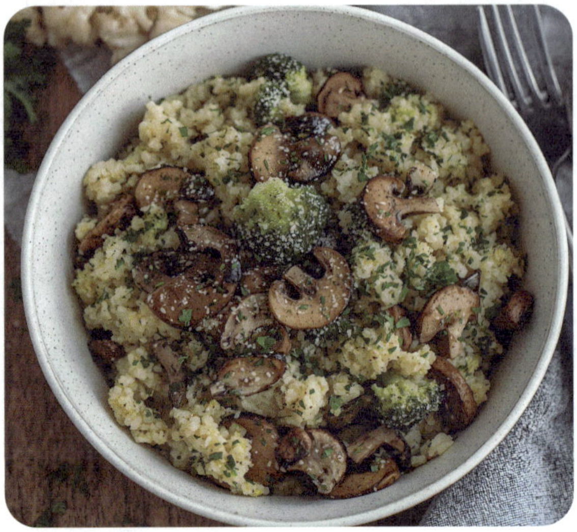

Servings	Prep time	Cook time
4	15 minutes	25 minutes

A creamy, earthy risotto made with broccoli rice and cauliflower rice, fragrant with garlic, mushrooms, and Parmesan. The technique is classic, but the ingredient swap keeps it low-carb and gluten-free.

INGREDIENTS

- 2 cups broccoli florets, processed or finely chopped ("riced")
- 2 cups cauliflower rice
- 8 oz cremini mushrooms, sliced
- 3 cloves garlic, minced
- ½ cup diced onion
- 4 cups gluten-free vegetable broth
- ¼ cup dry white wine (or additional broth)
- ½ cup grated Parmesan cheese
- 2 tbsp olive oil
- 2 tbsp butter
- Salt and black pepper
- Chopped parsley for garnish

DIRECTIONS

1. Heat olive oil in a large skillet. Sauté onion and garlic until fragrant, about 3 minutes.
2. Add mushrooms; cook until golden and moisture is released, about 6 minutes.
3. Stir in broccoli and cauliflower rice, coating everything in oil.
4. Add wine and cook until mostly evaporated.
5. Add broth ½ cup at a time, stirring frequently and allowing liquid to be absorbed before adding more.
6. When "rice" is tender and creamy (about 20 min), remove from heat. Stir in butter, Parmesan, salt, and pepper.
7. Garnish with parsley and serve immediately.

NUTRITION

Per Serving: 210 calories, 10g protein, 15g carbohydrates, 12g fat, 4g fiber

STORAGE

Best enjoyed fresh; leftovers keep for 2 days in the refrigerator.

Shrimp and Edamame Fried Rice

This Asian-inspired dish uses a 50/50 blend of cauliflower rice and green peas for extra color and sweetness. The shrimp are tossed with garlic, ginger, and a touch of peanut butter for richness—no added sugar, but tons of flavor.

Servings	Prep time	Cook time
4	10 minutes	15 minutes

INGREDIENTS

- 2 cups cauliflower rice
- 2 cups shelled edamame (fresh or thawed frozen)
- 12 oz large shrimp, peeled and deveined
- 2 eggs, beaten
- 3 green onions, sliced
- 2 cloves garlic, minced
- 1-inch ginger, grated
- 2 tbsp coconut oil
- 2 tbsp gluten-free soy sauce (or tamari)
- 1 tbsp natural peanut butter
- 1 tsp lime juice
- Salt and white pepper
- Chopped cilantro and lime wedges for serving

DIRECTIONS

1. Heat 1 tbsp coconut oil in a large skillet or wok. Stir-fry eggs quickly, breaking into small bits; remove and set aside.
2. In the same pan, heat remaining oil. Add shrimp, edamame, garlic, and ginger; stir-fry 2 min until shrimp turn pink.
3. Add cauliflower rice; stir-fry 3–4 min until vegetables are crisp-tender.
4. Return eggs to pan. Add soy sauce, peanut butter, lime juice, salt, and white pepper; toss to combine.
5. Stir in green onions and cook 1 min more.
6. Serve hot, garnished with cilantro and lime wedges.

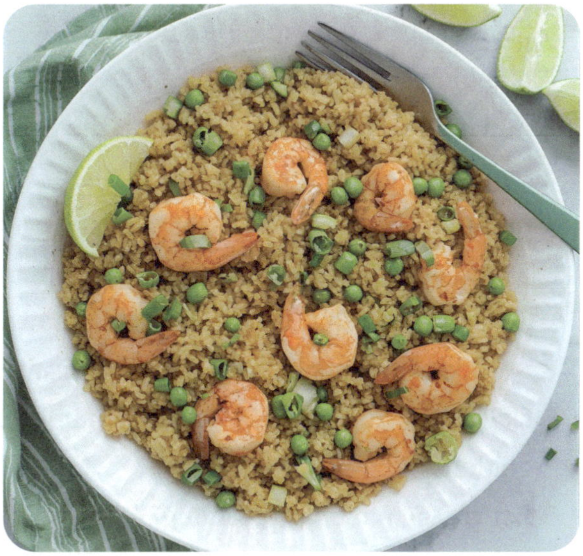

NUTRITION

Per serving: 280 calories, 25g protein, 18g carbohydrates, 12g fat, 5g fiber

STORAGE

Best eaten fresh, but keeps for 2 days refrigerated.

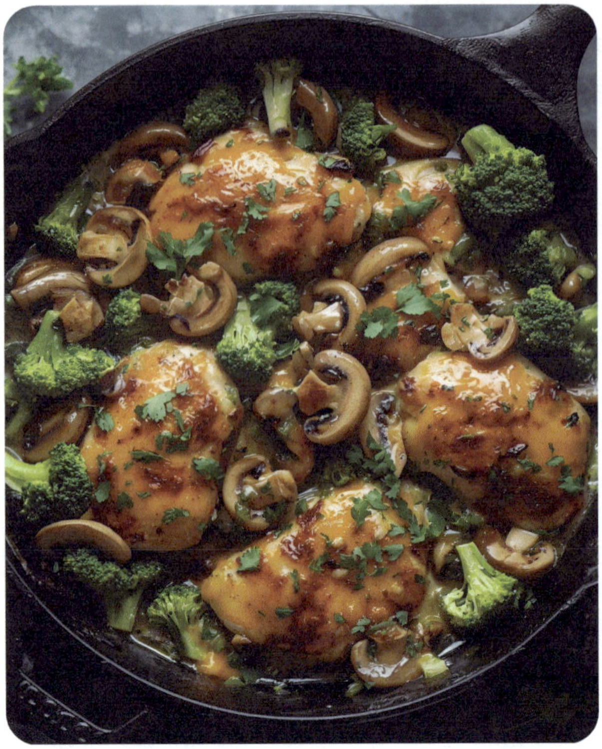

Cheesy Chicken and Broccoli Skillet

A creamy, comforting skillet dinner with tender chicken, broccoli rice, mushrooms, and a golden cheese crust—pure American comfort, gluten-free.

Servings	Prep time	Cook time
6	20 minutes	30 minutes

INGREDIENTS

- 2 lbs boneless, skinless chicken thighs, diced
- 4 cups broccoli rice (processed or finely chopped broccoli)
- 1 cup cauliflower rice (optional for bulk)
- 8 oz mushrooms, sliced
- 1 onion, diced
- 2 cups shredded cheddar cheese (or dairy-free cheese)
- 1 cup gluten-free chicken broth
- ¼ cup almond flour (for thickening)
- 2 tbsp olive oil
- 2 tbsp butter
- Salt, pepper, and garlic powder

DIRECTION

1. Preheat oven to 375°F (190°C).
2. In a large oven-safe skillet, sauté chicken until browned; remove and set aside.
3. In the same skillet, add butter and sauté onion and mushrooms for 5 min.
4. Stir in broccoli and cauliflower rice; cook 3 min.
5. Sprinkle with almond flour, stirring to combine.
6. Add broth and return chicken to the pan. Simmer until slightly thickened, about 5 minutes.
7. Stir in cheese, reserving a little for topping. Season with salt, pepper, and garlic powder.
8. Sprinkle remaining cheese on top. Transfer skillet to oven; bake 10 min until bubbly and golden.
9. Let rest 5 min before serving.

NUTRITION

Per serving: 340 calories, 30g protein, 10g carbohydrates, 18g fat, 4g fiber

STORAGE

Keeps refrigerated for up to 5 days or frozen for 2 months.

Smokey Beef and Cauliflower Skillet

6	15 minutes	20 minutes

A flavorful, low-carb skillet meal with all the satisfying flavors of Mexican cuisine.

DIRECTIONS

1. Heat large skillet over medium-high heat. Cook ground beef until browned, breaking up with spoon, about 8 minutes. Remove and drain excess fat.
2. Add olive oil to same skillet. Cook onion and bell pepper until softened, about 6 minutes.
3. Add garlic and cook 1 minute until fragrant.
4. Add cauliflower rice, diced tomatoes, green chiles, chili powder, cumin, smoked paprika, oregano, and cayenne. Cook 8-10 minutes until cauliflower is tender.
5. Return beef to skillet and stir to combine. Season with salt and pepper.
6. Top with cheese and cover until melted, about 2 minutes.
7. Garnish with cilantro and serve with avocado slices and lime wedges.

NUTRITION

Per serving: 335 calories, 26g protein, 10g carbohydrates, 22g fat, 4g fiber

STORAGE

Keeps for up to 3 days refrigerated. Reheat in skillet over medium heat.

INGREDIENTS

- 1 1/2 lbs ground beef (85/15)
- 1 large head cauliflower, riced (about 4 cups)
- 1 bell pepper, diced
- 1 medium onion, diced
- 3 cloves garlic, minced
- 1 can (14.5 oz) diced tomatoes, drained
- 1 can (4 oz) diced green chiles
- 2 tablespoons olive oil
- 2 teaspoons chili powder
- 1 teaspoon ground cumin
- 1 teaspoon smoked paprika
- 1/2 teaspoon oregano
- 1/4 teaspoon cayenne pepper
- 1 cup shredded Mexican cheese blend
- 1/4 cup fresh cilantro, chopped
- Salt and black pepper to taste
- Avocado slices and lime wedges for serving

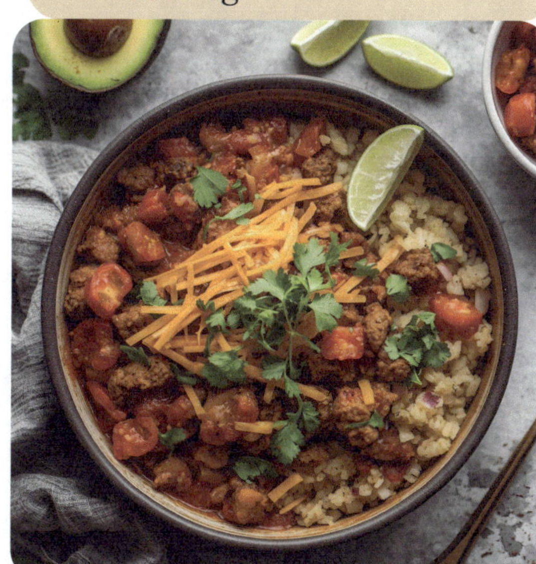

4

15 minutes

15 minutes

Tex-Mex Cauliflower & Black Bean Rice Bowl

A Tex-Mex-inspired bowl with spiced cauliflower rice, black beans, corn, and fresh toppings—bright, satisfying, and plant-forward.

INGREDIENTS

- 4 cups cauliflower rice
- 1 can (15 oz) black beans, rinsed
- 1 cup corn kernels (fresh or thawed)
- 1 red bell pepper, diced
- ½ red onion, diced
- 2 cloves garlic, minced
- 2 tbsp olive oil
- 1 tbsp chili powder
- 1 tsp ground cumin
- Salt and black pepper
- Juice of 1 lime
- Fresh cilantro, diced avocado, and lime wedges for serving

NUTRITION

Per serving: 290 calories, 12g protein, 42g carbohydrates, 9g fat, 12g fiber

STORAGE

Keeps refrigerated for up to 3 days.

DIRECTIONS

1. Heat oil in a large skillet. Sauté onion, bell pepper, and garlic until softened, about 5 min.
2. Add cauliflower rice, black beans, corn, chili powder, cumin, salt, and pepper. Stir-fry 5–7 min until cauliflower is tender.
3. Squeeze lime juice over everything and toss to combine.
4. Serve hot, topped with cilantro, avocado, and extra lime.

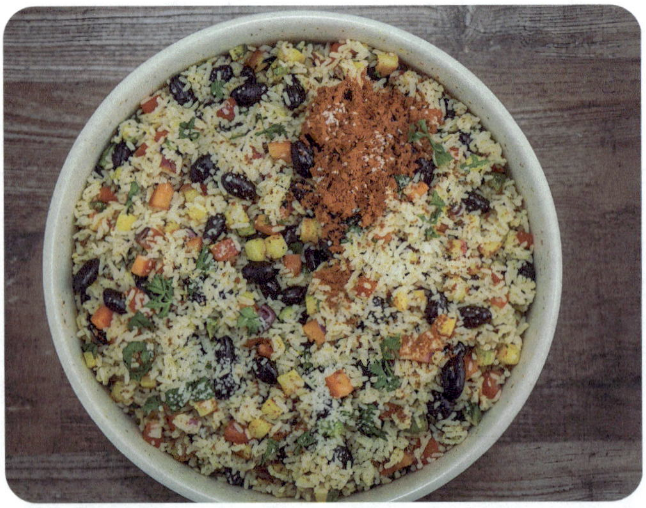

Lemon-Herb Cauliflower & Quinoa Pilaf

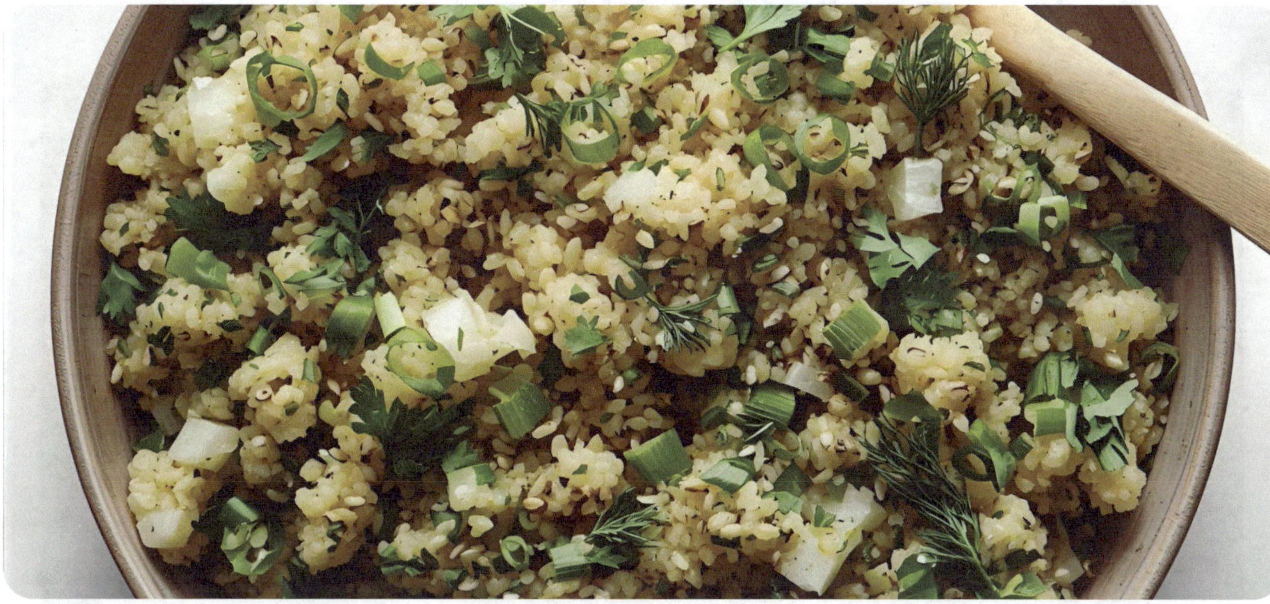

6 | 15 minutes | 20 minutes

A fresh, zesty pilaf blending cauliflower rice, quinoa, and bright garden herbs.

INGREDIENTS

- 3 cups cauliflower rice
- 1½ cups cooked quinoa (certified gluten-free)
- 4 green onions, sliced
- ¼ cup chopped fresh parsley
- ¼ cup chopped fresh dill
- Zest and juice of 1 lemon
- 3 tbsp olive oil
- Salt and black pepper
- ¼ cup toasted almonds or pine nuts (optional)

DIRECTIONS

1. Heat olive oil in a large skillet over medium heat. Add cauliflower rice and sauté until just tender, about 5 minutes.
2. Stir in cooked quinoa, green onions, parsley, dill, lemon zest, lemon juice, salt, and pepper.
3. Cook, stirring occasionally, for 2–3 minutes more until everything is heated through and the flavors are well blended.
4. Transfer to a serving dish and sprinkle with toasted nuts if desired.

NUTRITION

Per serving: 210 calories, 6g protein, 25g carbohydrates, 10g fat, 6g fiber

STORAGE

Keeps refrigerated for up to 5 days.

Coconut-Curry Shrimp with Green Beans & Cauliflower Rice

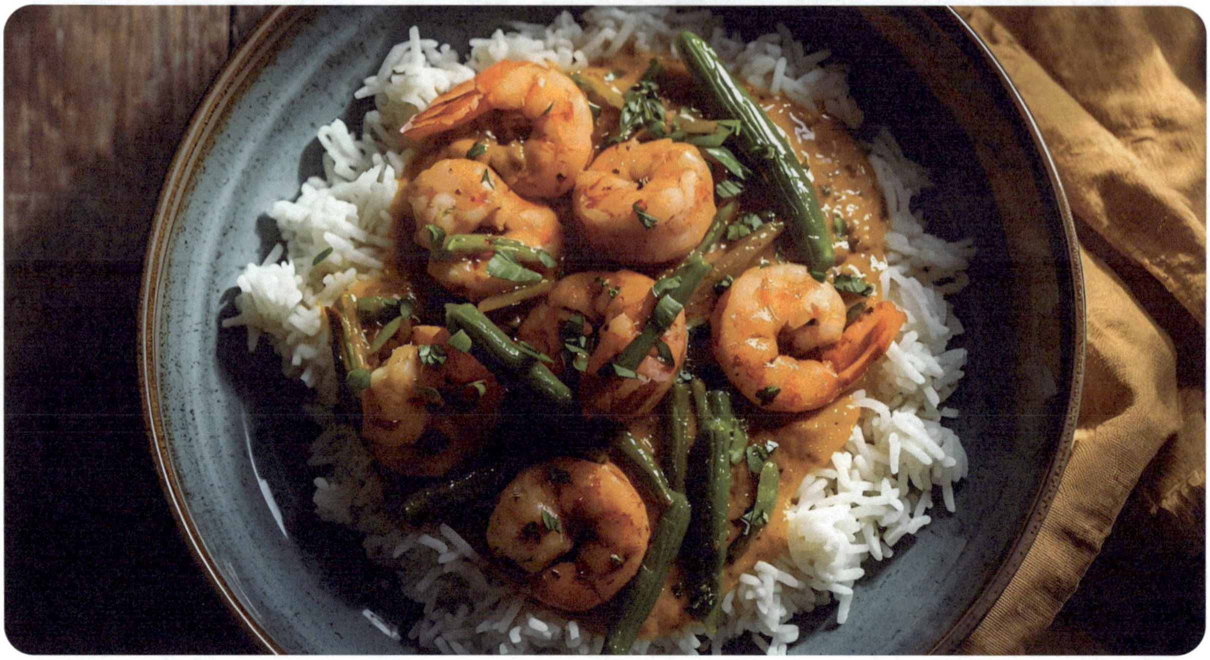

Shrimp and green beans simmered in creamy coconut curry, served over jasmine rice.

Servings	Prep time	Cook time
4	10 minutes	20 minutes

INGREDIENTS

- 1 lb large shrimp, peeled and deveined
- 1 lb green beans, trimmed
- 1 can (14 oz) lite coconut milk
- 2 tbsp gluten-free red curry paste
- 1 tbsp fish sauce
- 1 tsp erythritol (or sweetener of choice)
- 2 cloves garlic, minced
- 1 tbsp fresh lime juice
- Fresh cilantro and lime wedges for garnish
- Steamed cauliflower rice

DIRECTIONS

1. Steam green beans until crisp-tender; set aside.
2. In a skillet, sauté garlic in a bit of coconut oil until fragrant.
3. Add curry paste, coconut milk, fish sauce, and sweetener; simmer 5 min.
4. Stir in shrimp and green beans; simmer 3–5 min until shrimp are pink.
5. Finish with lime juice, cilantro, and more lime wedges. Serve over rice.

NUTRITION

Per serving with half cup rice bar: 320 calories, 22g protein, 36g carbohydrates, 10g fat, 4g fiber

STORAGE

Best served fresh, but keeps 2 days refrigerated.

4	10 minutes	15 minutes

Pesto Shrimp "Pasotto"

This colorful, protein-packed meal brings together tender shrimp, earthy mushrooms, and sweet grape tomatoes tossed in a vibrant basil pesto. The chickpea orzo adds a subtle nutty flavor and extra fiber for blood sugar-friendly satisfaction. When it comes together, it feels like a cross between pasta and risotto, I nicknamed it Pasotto!

INGREDIENTS

- 8 oz chickpea orzo pasta
- 1 lb shrimp, peeled and deveined
- 2 tbsp olive oil, divided
- 2 cups baby bella mushrooms, sliced
- 1 cup grape tomatoes, halved
- 2 cloves garlic, minced
- ¼ cup prepared basil pesto (store-bought or homemade, no added sugar)
- 2 tbsp grated Parmesan cheese (optional)
- Salt and pepper to taste
- Fresh basil leaves for garnish

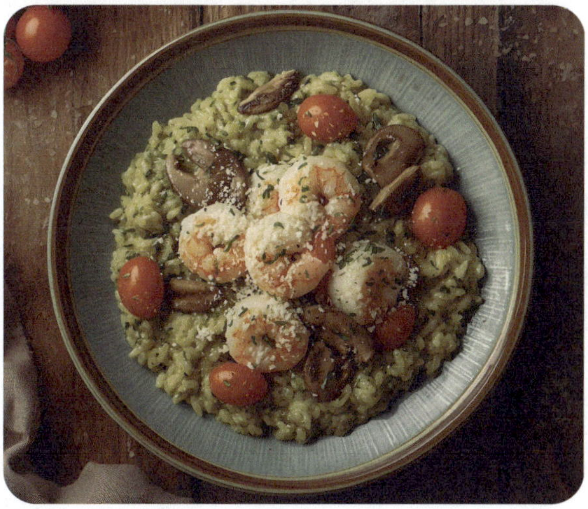

DIRECTIONS

1. Bring a large pot of salted water to a gentle boil. Cook chickpea orzo just until al dente, about 6–7 minutes. Drain and set aside, reserving ¼ cup cooking water.
2. In a large skillet, heat 1 tbsp olive oil over medium heat. Add mushrooms and cook 4 minutes until browned. Add tomatoes and garlic; sauté 2 minutes until softened.
3. Push vegetables to the side, add remaining 1 tbsp olive oil, and toss in shrimp. Cook 2–3 minutes per side until pink and opaque.
4. Reduce heat to low. Add cooked orzo and pesto to the pan, tossing gently. Add a splash of reserved pasta water to loosen the sauce if needed.
5. Season with salt and pepper. Sprinkle with Parmesan and garnish with fresh basil. Serve warm.

NUTRITION

Per serving: 365 calories, 32g protein, 18g carbohydrates, 18g fat, 5g fiber

STORAGE

Keeps refrigerated for up to 3 days.

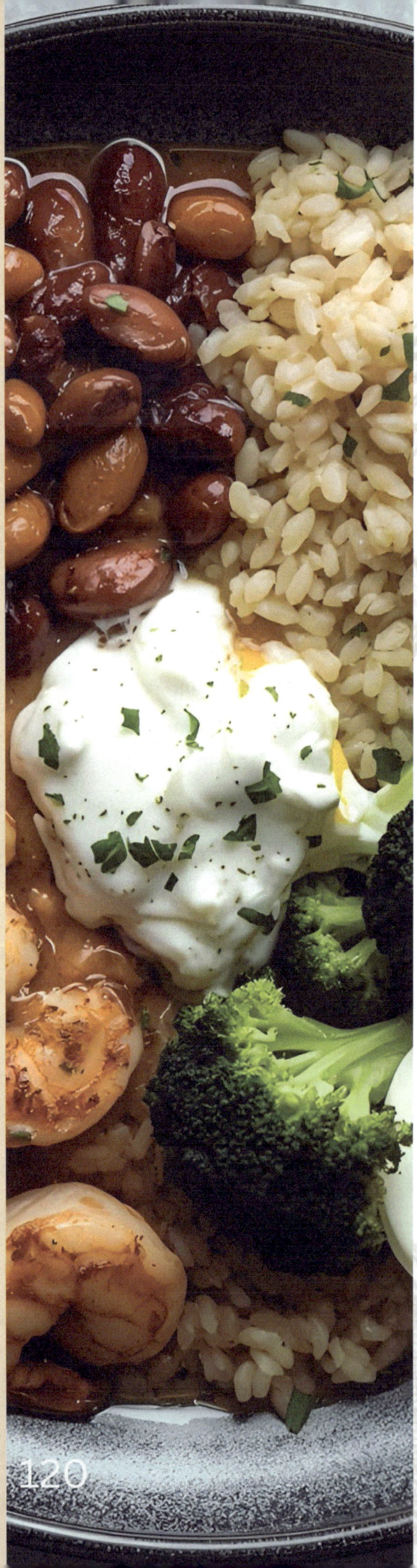

Why These Recipes Work

Diverse Protein Sources: Chicken, shrimp, beans, and eggs make frequent appearances, supporting blood sugar stability and appealing to varied tastes.

Low-Glycemic Carbs: Cauliflower, broccoli, and farro provide fiber and texture without spiking glucose.

Gluten-Free by Design: No wheat, barley, or rye; only gluten-free grains and whole-food substitutions.

American & Global Flavors: From Cajun to Tex-Mex to Mediterranean, each dish is familiar yet fresh.

Meal-Prep Friendly: All recipes can be made ahead, frozen, or repurposed for lunches.

Nutritional Balance: High fiber, moderate protein, and healthy fats—key for diabetes and celiac management.

CHAPTER 11

Pasta Perfecto!

List of Recipes

1. Thick Italian Bolognese
2. Hearts of Palm Spinach Lasagne
3. Vodka Sauce with Shrimp on Zucchini Noodles
4. Clam Sauce with Hearts of Palm
5. Shirataki Noodles with Pomodoro
6. Eggplant Lasagne with Red Sauce
7. Chicken Alfredo
8. Shirataki with Pesto Side Dish
9. Beef Stroganoff with Zucchini Noodles
10. Rice Pasta Macaroni and Cheese

Pasta night doesn't have to become a distant memory when you're managing both celiac disease and diabetes. In fact, this chapter will show you how to create even more satisfying, nutritious, and delicious "pasta" meals than you ever enjoyed before. The secret lies in understanding that pasta has always been about more than wheat—it's about texture, sauce delivery, comfort, and bringing people together around the table.

Traditional wheat pasta poses a double challenge for those of us in the celiabetic community. Not only does it contain gluten that damages our intestinal villi, but its high glycemic impact can send blood sugar soaring within minutes of eating. The wonderful news is that once you discover the incredible variety of pasta alternatives available today, you'll wonder why anyone limits themselves to plain wheat noodles.

This chapter presents a comprehensive guide to pasta substitutes that range from virtually zero-carb vegetable noodles to protein-rich legume pastas that actually improve your meal's nutritional profile. You'll learn how to spiralize zucchini without ending up with mushy noodles, which store-bought alternatives are worth your money, and how to pair each pasta type with the sauces that complement it best. Some of these alternatives will surprise you with how closely they mimic traditional pasta, while others will win you over with unique textures and flavors that create entirely new favorite dishes.

We'll explore cooking techniques specific to each pasta type—because gluten-free pasta behaves differently than wheat pasta and requires different timing, water ratios, and handling. You'll discover how to prevent the dreaded gummy texture, achieve perfect al dente bite, and keep your pasta from clumping or falling apart.

Beyond the pasta itself, this chapter includes complete meal solutions with perfectly paired sauces, protein additions, and vegetable combinations that create balanced, blood sugar-friendly dinners. Each recipe includes glycemic impact ratings and strategies for portion control without feeling deprived.

At the end of this chapter, you'll find reference pages with detailed comparison charts of pasta alternatives, cooking time guides, nutritional breakdowns, and troubleshooting solutions for common pasta problems. These quick-reference resources will become your go-to guides for confident pasta preparation every time.

Thick Italian Bolognese

A rich, hearty meat sauce so thick and satisfying that pasta becomes optional. Perfect over zucchini noodles, gluten free gnocchi, or enjoyed on its own with crusty gluten-free bread. I make a double or triple batch and freeze it for easy weeknight meals.

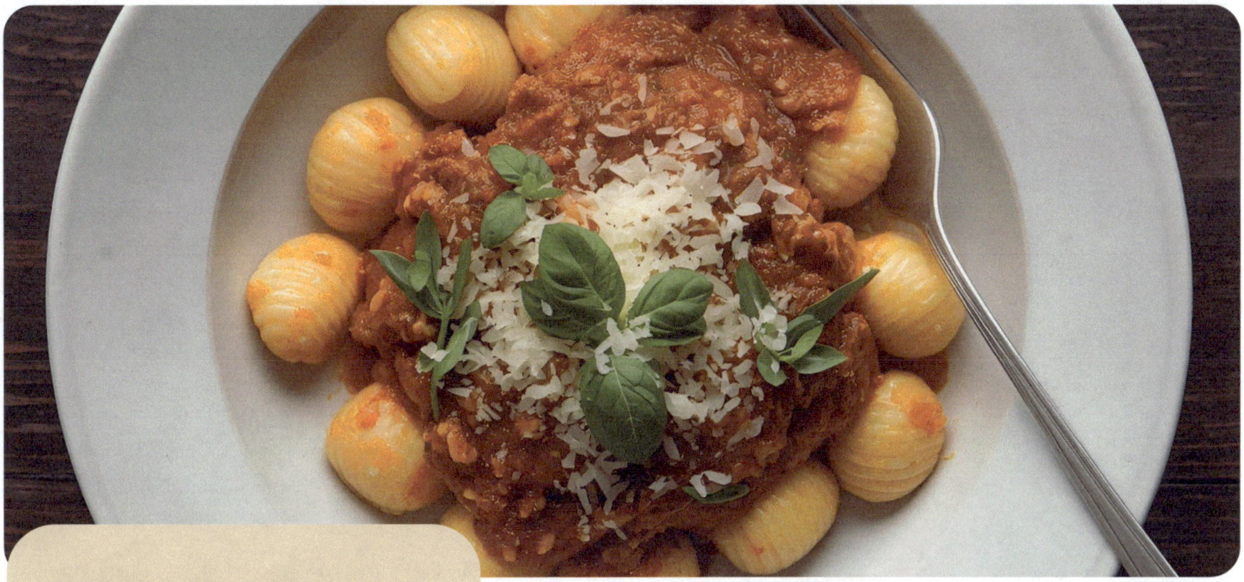

INGREDIENTS

- 2 lbs ground beef (80/20)
- 1 lb ground pork
- 2 tablespoons olive oil
- 1 large onion, finely diced
- 2 large carrots, finely diced
- 2 stalks celery, finely diced
- 6 cloves garlic, minced
- 1 can (6 oz) tomato paste
- 1 cup dry white wine
- 1 can (28 oz) crushed tomatoes
- 1 can (14 oz) diced tomatoes
- 2 cups chicken broth
- 1 cup whole milk
- 2 tablespoons fresh basil, chopped
- 1 tablespoon fresh oregano
- 2 bay leaves
- 1 teaspoon salt
- 1/2 teaspoon black pepper
- 1 rind from a parmesan wedge

8	25 minutes	4 hr 30 min

DIRECTIONS

1. Heat olive oil in large heavy-bottomed pot over medium-high heat.
2. Brown ground beef and pork in batches, breaking up with spoon, about 8 minutes per batch. Remove meat and set aside.
3. In same pot, sauté onion, carrots, and celery until softened, about 8 minutes.
4. Add garlic and cook 1 minute until fragrant.
5. Stir in tomato paste and cook 3 minutes until darkened.
6. Add wine and scrape up browned bits from bottom of pot.
7. Return meat to pot and add crushed tomatoes, diced tomatoes, chicken broth, milk, cheese rind, basil, oregano, bay leaves, salt, and pepper.
8. Bring to boil, then reduce heat to low and simmer uncovered 4 to 6 hours, stirring occasionally.
9. Remove bay leaves and cheese rind before serving.

NUTRITION

Per serving: 425 calories, 32g protein, 12g carbohydrates, 28g fat, 3g fiber

STORAGE

Keeps refrigerated for 5 days. Freezes for up to 3 months. Reheat gently, adding broth if needed.

Hearts of Palm Spinach Lasagne

8 | 20 minutes | 45 minutes

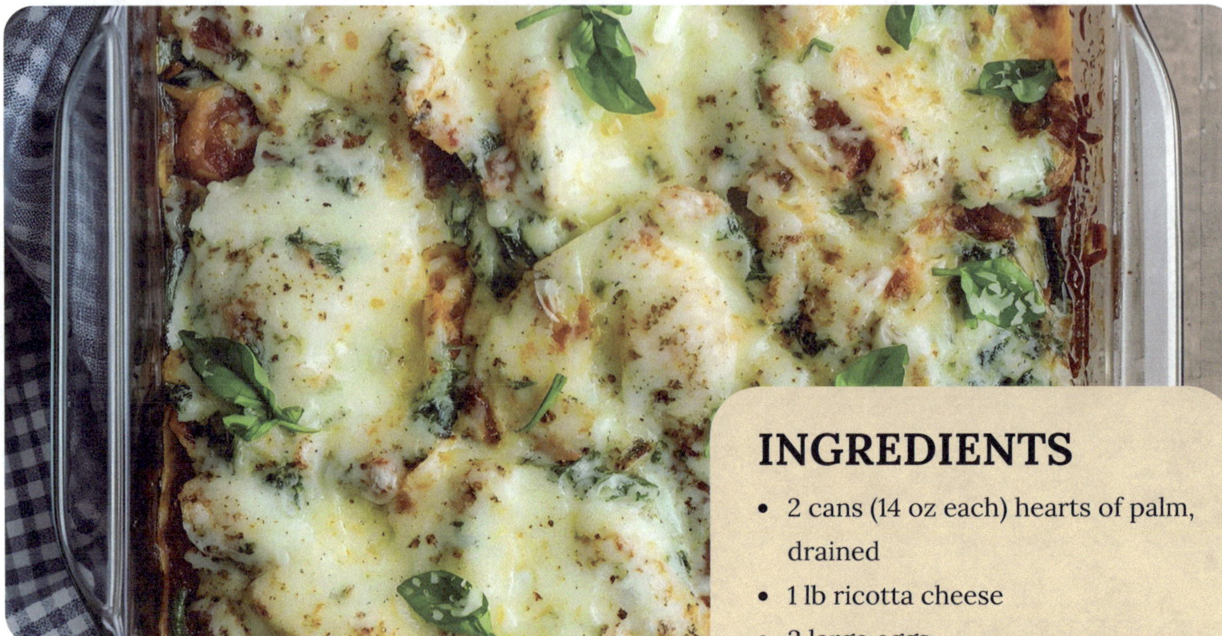

A sophisticated vegetarian lasagne using hearts of palm as noodles and packed with nutrient-rich spinach and creamy ricotta.

INGREDIENTS

- 2 cans (14 oz each) hearts of palm, drained
- 1 lb ricotta cheese
- 2 large eggs
- 10 oz fresh spinach, chopped
- 3 cups mozzarella cheese, shredded
- 1 cup Parmesan cheese, grated
- 3 cups marinara sauce (sugar-free)
- 3 cloves garlic, minced
- 1/4 cup fresh basil, chopped
- 2 tablespoons olive oil
- 1 teaspoon salt
- 1/2 teaspoon black pepper
- 1/4 teaspoon nutmeg

DIRECTIONS

1. Preheat oven to 375°F (190°C). Grease 9x13-inch baking dish.
2. Slice hearts of palm lengthwise into thin, flat sheets resembling lasagne noodles. (You can find premade online.)
3. Heat olive oil in large skillet and sauté spinach until wilted, about 3 minutes. Cool and squeeze out excess moisture.
4. In bowl, combine ricotta, eggs, cooked spinach, garlic, basil, salt, pepper, and nutmeg.
5. Spread 1/2 cup marinara in bottom of prepared dish.
6. Layer 1/3 of hearts of palm, 1/2 ricotta mixture, 1 cup mozzarella, and 1 cup marinara.
7. Repeat layers, ending with remaining hearts of palm, marinara, mozzarella, and Parmesan.
8. Cover with foil and bake 30 minutes.
9. Remove foil and bake 15 minutes until bubbly and golden.
10. Let rest 10 minutes before serving.

NUTRITION

Per serving: 285 calories, 22g protein, 12g carbohydrates, 18g fat, 4g fiber

STORAGE

Refrigerate up to 3 days. Can be assembled 1 day ahead before baking

Vodka Sauce with Shrimp on Zucchini Noodles

6 | 15 minutes | 20 minutes

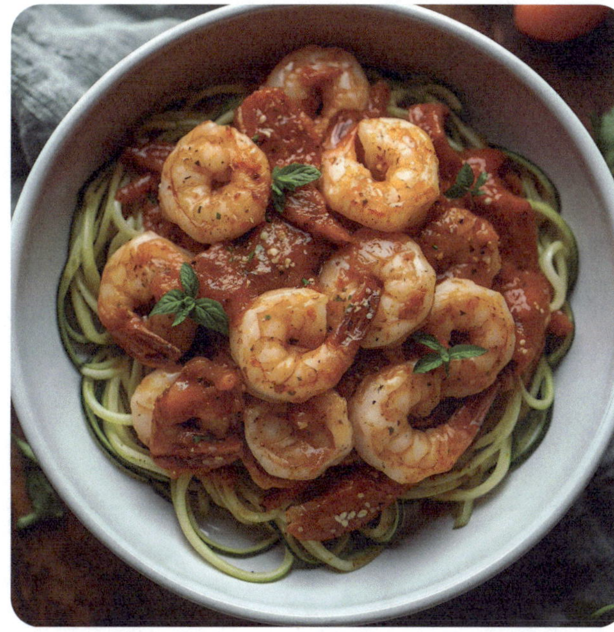

Creamy, tomato-based vodka sauce with succulent shrimp served over fresh zucchini noodles for an elegant, low-carb dinner.

INGREDIENTS

- 1 1/2 lbs large shrimp, peeled and deveined
- 4 large zucchini, spiralized
- 3 tablespoons olive oil
- 1 small onion, finely diced
- 4 cloves garlic, minced
- 1/2 cup vodka
- 1 can (14 oz) crushed tomatoes
- 1/2 cup heavy cream
- 1/4 cup fresh basil, chopped
- 2 tablespoons fresh parsley, chopped
- 1 teaspoon salt
- 1/2 teaspoon black pepper
- 1/4 teaspoon red pepper flakes
- 2 tablespoons butter

DIRECTIONS

1. Spiralize zucchini and salt lightly. Let drain in colander 15 minutes, then pat dry.
2. Season shrimp with salt and pepper.
3. Heat 2 tablespoons olive oil in large skillet over medium-high heat. Cook shrimp 2-3 minutes per side until pink. Remove and set aside.
4. In same skillet, heat remaining oil and sauté onion until softened, about 5 minutes.
5. Add garlic and cook 1 minute.
6. Add vodka and cook 2 minutes to burn off alcohol.
7. Add crushed tomatoes, salt, pepper, and red pepper flakes. Simmer 10 minutes.
8. Stir in cream and cook 2 minutes until heated through.
9. Return shrimp to pan and add butter, basil, and parsley.
10. Quickly sauté zucchini noodles in separate pan 1-2 minutes, then serve topped with shrimp and sauce.

NUTRITION

Per serving: 295 calories, 26g protein, 10g carbohydrates, 16g fat, 3g fiber

STORAGE

Best served immediately. Sauce can be made 1 day ahead and reheated.

Clam Sauce with Hearts of Palm

Classic white clam sauce featuring tender hearts of palm as a sophisticated pasta substitute with briny, garlicky flavors.

Servings	Prep time	Cook time
4	10 minutes	15 minutes

DIRECTION

1. Gently separate hearts of palm into linguine-like strands with a fork. (You can find premade online.)
2. Drain clams, reserving 1/2 cup of juice.
3. Heat olive oil in large skillet over medium heat.
4. Add garlic and cook until fragrant and lightly golden, about 2 minutes.
5. Add wine and reserved clam juice. Simmer 3 minutes.
6. Add clams, red pepper flakes, salt, and pepper. Cook 2 minutes.
7. Add hearts of palm and gently toss to warm through, about 1 minute.
8. Remove from heat and stir in butter, parsley, lemon juice, and zest.
9. Serve immediately with additional parsley if desired.

INGREDIENTS

- 2 cans (14 oz each) hearts of palm, drained
- 3 cans (6.5 oz each) chopped clams, with juice
- 1/4 cup olive oil
- 6 cloves garlic, thinly sliced
- 1/2 cup dry white wine
- 1/4 cup fresh parsley, chopped
- 2 tablespoons fresh lemon juice
- 1 tablespoon lemon zest
- 1/4 teaspoon red pepper flakes
- 1/2 teaspoon salt
- 1/4 teaspoon black pepper
- 3 tablespoons butter

NUTRITION

Per serving: 245 calories, 18g protein, 8g carbohydrates, 16g fat, 2g fiber

STORAGE

Best served immediately. Does not store well due to delicate texture of hearts of palm.

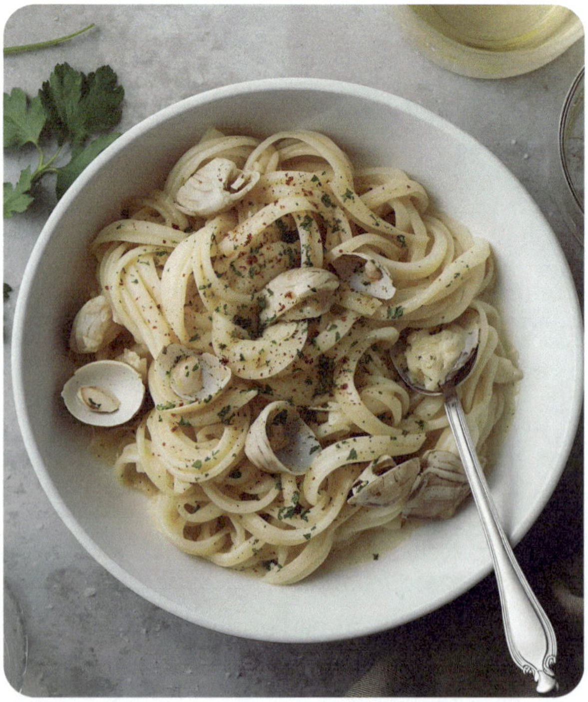

4

15 minutes

25 minutes

Shirataki Noodles with Pomodoro

Simple, fresh tomato sauce with aromatic herbs served over shirataki noodles for a virtually carb-free Italian classic.

INGREDIENTS

- 2 packages (8 oz each) shirataki fettuccine
- 2 lbs ripe tomatoes, peeled and chopped
- 1/4 cup olive oil
- 4 cloves garlic, minced
- 1/4 cup fresh basil, chopped
- 2 tablespoons fresh oregano
- 1 teaspoon salt
- 1/2 teaspoon black pepper
- 1/4 cup Parmesan cheese, grated
- 2 tablespoons fresh parsley, chopped

DIRECTIONS

1. Rinse shirataki noodles thoroughly under cold water for 2 minutes. Dry-roast in hot pan for 2 minutes to improve texture. Set aside.
2. To peel tomatoes: Score X on bottom, blanch in boiling water 30 seconds, transfer to ice water, then slip off skins.
3. Heat olive oil in large skillet over medium heat.
4. Add garlic and cook until fragrant, about 1 minute.
5. Add chopped tomatoes, salt, and pepper. Cook 15 minutes, stirring occasionally.
6. Stir in basil and oregano. Cook 5 minutes more.
7. Add prepared shirataki noodles and toss to warm through, about 2 minutes.
8. Serve topped with Parmesan and fresh parsley.

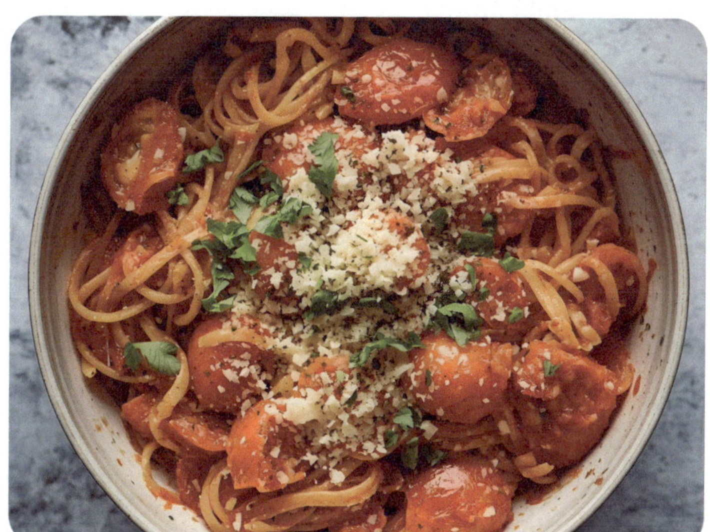

NUTRITION

Per serving: 155 calories, 4g protein, 12g carbohydrates, 12g fat, 4g fiber

STORAGE

Sauce keeps refrigerated for 3 days. Best to prepare fresh shirataki when serving.

Eggplant Lasagne with Red Sauce

8 | 30 minutes | 1 hr 15 min

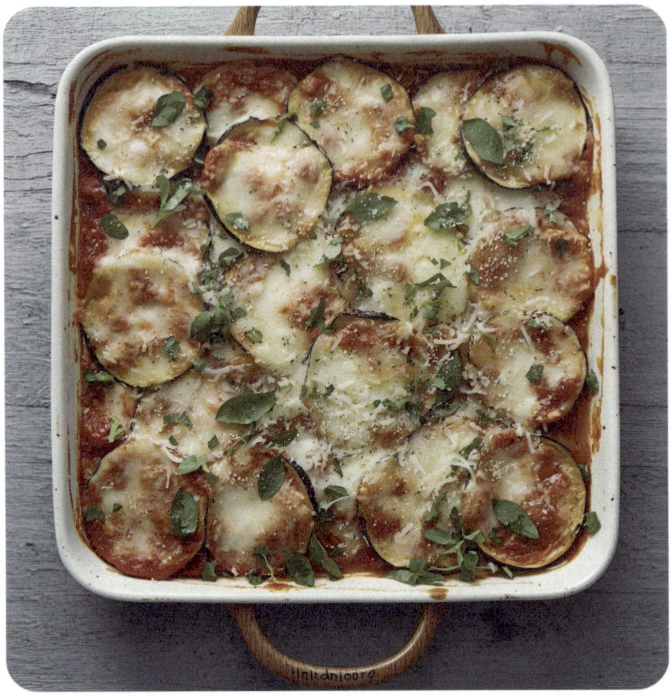

Hearty, satisfying lasagne using roasted eggplant slices instead of pasta, layered with rich meat sauce and creamy cheese.

INGREDIENTS

- 2 large eggplants, sliced lengthwise 1/4-inch thick
- 1 lb ground beef
- 3 cups marinara sauce (sugar-free)
- 1 lb ricotta cheese
- 2 large eggs
- 2 cups mozzarella cheese, shredded
- 1/2 cup Parmesan cheese, grated
- 1/4 cup fresh basil, chopped
- 3 cloves garlic, minced
- 1/4 cup olive oil
- 2 teaspoons salt
- 1 teaspoon black pepper
- 1 teaspoon Italian seasoning

DIRECTIONS

1. Preheat oven to 400°F (200°C). Salt eggplant slices and let drain 20 minutes. Pat dry.
2. Brush eggplant with olive oil and roast on baking sheets 20 minutes until tender.
3. Brown ground beef in large skillet, breaking up with spoon. Drain fat.
4. Add 2 cups marinara sauce to beef and simmer 10 minutes.
5. In bowl, combine ricotta, eggs, garlic, basil, 1 teaspoon salt, and 1/2 teaspoon pepper.
6. Reduce oven to 375°F (190°C). Grease 9x13-inch baking dish.
7. Layer 1/2 cup marinara in dish, then 1/3 eggplant, 1/2 ricotta mixture, 1/2 meat sauce, 1/3 mozzarella.
8. Repeat layers, ending with eggplant, remaining marinara, mozzarella, and Parmesan.
9. Cover and bake 30 minutes. Uncover and bake 15 minutes until bubbly.
10. Let rest 15 minutes before serving.

NUTRITION

Per serving: 385 calories, 28g protein, 16g carbohydrates, 24g fat, 6g fiber

STORAGE

Refrigerate up to 4 days. Can be assembled 1 day ahead before baking.

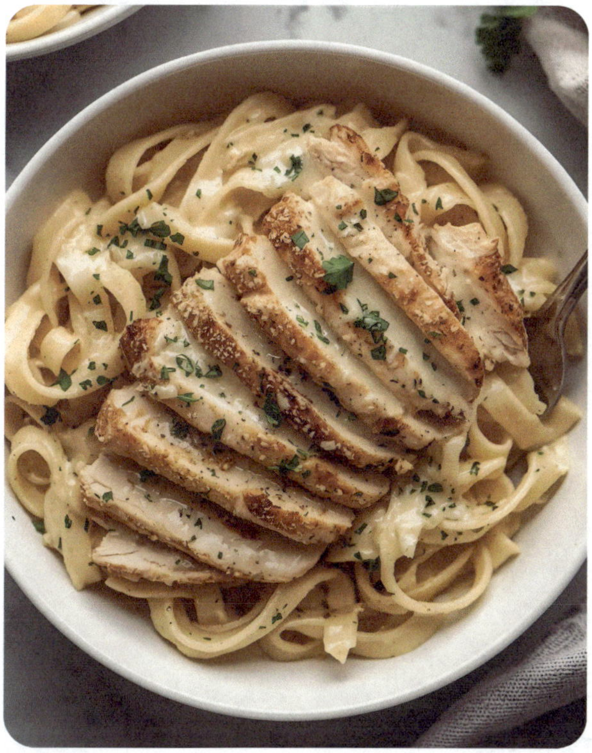

Chicken Alfredo

Creamy, rich Alfredo sauce with tender chicken served over your choice of gluten-free pasta alternative for ultimate comfort food satisfaction

Servings	Prep time	Cook time
6	15 minutes	25 minutes

NUTRITION

Per serving: 565 calories, 35g protein, 8g carbohydrates, 44g fat, 2g fiber

STORAGE

Sauce is best served immediately but can be gently reheated with additional cream if needed.

INGREDIENTS

- 1 1/2 lbs boneless, skinless chicken breasts, sliced
- 8 oz gluten-free fettuccine or 4 large zucchini, spiralized
- 1/2 cup butter
- 4 cloves garlic, minced
- 1 1/2 cups heavy cream
- 1 1/2 cups Parmesan cheese, freshly grated
- 1/4 cup fresh parsley, chopped
- 3 tablespoons olive oil
- 1 teaspoon salt
- 1/2 teaspoon black pepper
- 1/4 teaspoon nutmeg

DIRECTIONS

1. If using zucchini, spiralize and salt lightly. Let drain 15 minutes, then pat dry. If using gluten-free pasta, cook according to package directions.
2. Season chicken with salt and pepper.
3. Heat olive oil in large skillet over medium-high heat. Cook chicken 6-7 minutes per side until golden and cooked through. Remove and slice.
4. In same skillet, melt butter over medium heat. Add garlic and cook 1 minute.
5. Gradually whisk in cream and bring to gentle simmer.
6. Remove from heat and gradually whisk in Parmesan cheese until smooth.
7. Season with salt, pepper, and nutmeg.
8. If using zucchini noodles, quickly sauté 1-2 minutes until just warmed.
9. Toss pasta or zucchini with Alfredo sauce, add sliced chicken, and garnish with parsley.

Shirataki with Pesto Side Dish

Light, herbal pesto tossed with shirataki noodles creates the perfect low-carb side dish to complement any protein-centered meal.

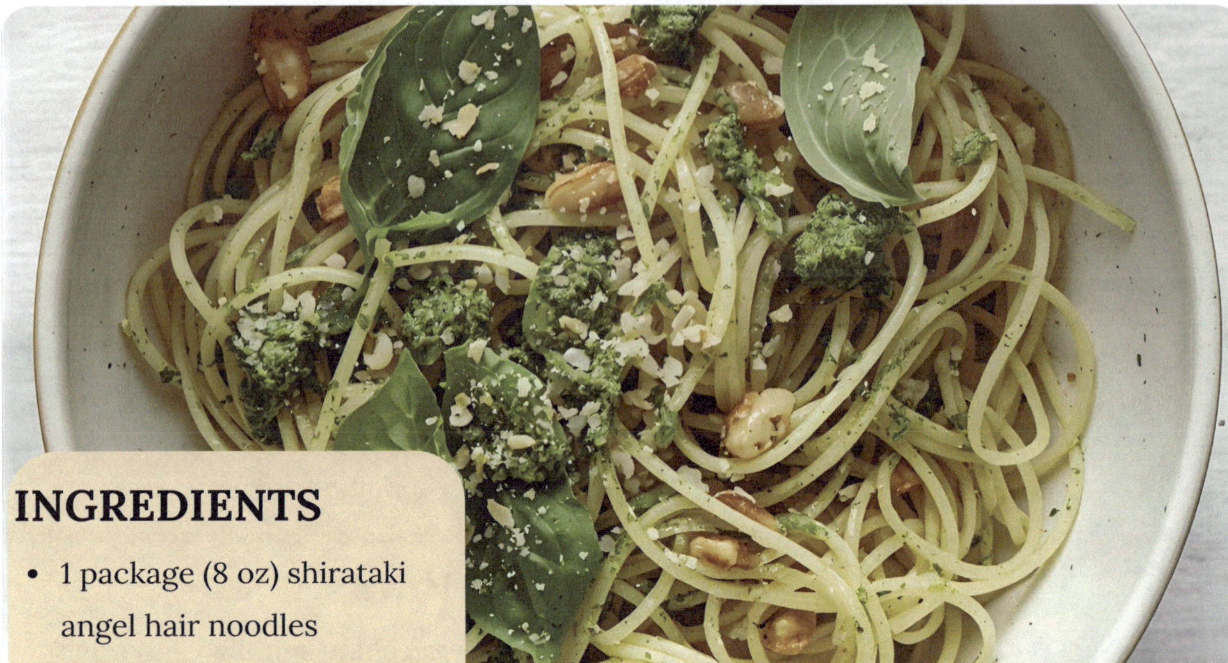

INGREDIENTS

- 1 package (8 oz) shirataki angel hair noodles
- 2 cups fresh basil leaves
- 1/2 cup pine nuts, toasted
- 3 cloves garlic
- 1/2 cup Parmesan cheese, grated
- 1/2 cup olive oil
- 1 tablespoon lemon juice
- 1/2 teaspoon salt
- 1/4 teaspoon black pepper

4 | 10 minutes | 5 minutes

DIRECTIONS

1. Rinse shirataki noodles thoroughly under cold water for 2 minutes. Dry-roast in hot pan for 2 minutes. Set aside.
2. Toast pine nuts in dry skillet over medium heat 3-4 minutes until golden. Cool completely.
3. In food processor, pulse garlic until minced.
4. Add basil, pine nuts, and salt. Pulse until chopped.
5. With processor running, slowly drizzle in olive oil until smooth paste forms.
6. Transfer to bowl and stir in Parmesan, lemon juice, and pepper.
7. Toss prepared shirataki noodles with pesto until well coated.
8. Serve at room temperature or slightly warmed.

NUTRITION

Per serving: 285 calories, 8g protein, 5g carbohydrates, 28g fat, 2g fiber

STORAGE

Pesto keeps refrigerated for 1 week. Best to toss with noodles just before serving.

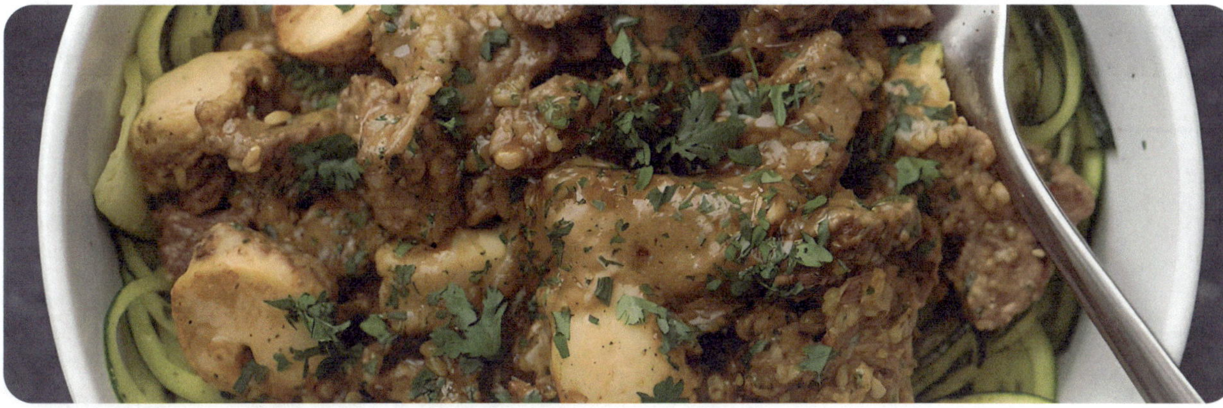

Beef Stroganoff with Zucchini Noodles

Servings	Prep time	Cook time
6	15 minutes	25 minutes

Rich, creamy beef stroganoff served over fresh zucchini noodles for a lighter take on this beloved comfort classic.

INGREDIENTS

- 2 lbs beef sirloin, cut into strips
- 3 tablespoons olive oil
- 1 large onion, sliced
- 12 oz mushrooms, sliced
- 3 cloves garlic, minced
- 2 tablespoons almond flour
- 2 cups beef broth
- 1 cup sour cream
- 2 tablespoons Dijon mustard
- 2 tablespoons fresh dill, chopped
- 4 large zucchini, spiralized
- Salt and black pepper to taste
- Fresh parsley for garnish

DIRECTIONS

1. Season beef strips with salt and pepper.
2. Heat 2 tablespoons olive oil in large skillet over medium-high heat. Brown beef in batches, about 6 minutes total. Remove and set aside.
3. Add remaining oil to same pan. Cook onion and mushrooms until golden, about 10 minutes.
4. Add garlic and cook 1 minute until fragrant.
5. Sprinkle almond flour over vegetables and cook 2 minutes, stirring constantly.
6. Gradually add beef broth, stirring until thickened, about 5 minutes.
7. Return beef to pan and simmer 5 minutes.
8. Remove from heat and stir in sour cream, Dijon mustard, and dill. Don't boil after adding sour cream.
9. Meanwhile, dry sauté zucchini noodles in large pan for 2-3 minutes until just tender.
10. Serve stroganoff over zucchini noodles, garnished with parsley.

NUTRITION

Per serving: 345 calories, 32g protein, 12g carbohydrates, 20g fat, 3g fiber

STORAGE

Stroganoff keeps for up to 3 days refrigerated. Prepare fresh zucchini noodles for best texture.

Rice Pasta Macaroni and Cheese

8 | 15 minutes | 25 minutes

Classic comfort food made with brown rice pasta and a rich, creamy cheese sauce that rivals any traditional mac and cheese.

DIRECTION

1. Cook rice pasta according to package directions until al dente. Drain and rinse briefly with cold water.
2. In large saucepan, melt butter over medium heat.
3. Whisk in almond flour and cook 2 minutes, stirring constantly.
4. Gradually whisk in milk until smooth. Cook, stirring frequently, until thickened, about 5 minutes.
5. Remove from heat and whisk in cream cheese until smooth.
6. Gradually stir in cheddar and Gruyere cheeses until melted.
7. Stir in Dijon mustard, garlic powder, salt, and pepper.
8. Add cooked pasta and stir until well coated.
9. Serve immediately, garnished with paprika and chives.","

INGREDIENTS

- 12 oz brown rice elbow macaroni
- 4 tablespoons butter
- 1/4 cup almond flour
- 2 1/2 cups whole milk
- 2 cups sharp cheddar cheese, shredded
- 1/2 cup Gruyere cheese, shredded
- 1/4 cup cream cheese, softened
- 1 teaspoon Dijon mustard
- 1/2 teaspoon garlic powder
- 1/2 teaspoon salt
- 1/4 teaspoon black pepper
- 1/4 teaspoon paprika
- 2 tablespoons chives, chopped

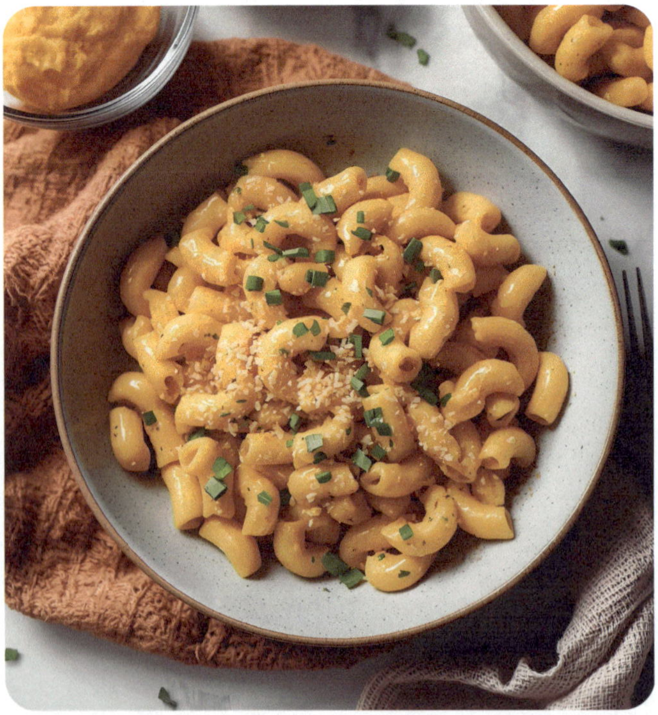

NUTRITION

Per serving: 385 calories, 16g protein, 42g carbohydrates, 18g fat, 2g fiber

STORAGE

Best served immediately. Leftovers keep 3 days refrigerated. Reheat with additional milk if needed.

Deep Dish Dive!

The Celiabetic Advantage: Better Than the Original

What I've discovered through years of recipe development and testing is that many pasta substitutes offer significant advantages over wheat pasta. Zucchini noodles provide hydration and potassium while delivering a satisfying al dente texture. Shirataki noodles allow you to enjoy generous portions without any blood sugar impact. Chickpea pasta delivers more protein than most chicken dishes while maintaining that satisfying pasta experience your family craves.

The key to success with pasta alternatives lies in understanding each one's unique properties and matching them with appropriate cooking techniques and sauces. A delicate hearts of palm linguine calls for different treatment than hearty lentil shells, just as angel hair pasta requires different handling than rigatoni. Once you master these relationships, you'll have complete freedom to recreate any pasta dish while supporting your health goals.

Building Your Alternative Pasta Pantry

Throughout this chapter, I'll guide you through the essential pasta alternatives to keep on hand, from the quick-cooking convenience of shirataki noodles to the make-ahead versatility of spiralized vegetables. You'll learn which alternatives work best for meal prep, which ones freeze successfully, and which deserve a permanent place in your pantry for emergency weeknight dinners.

More importantly, you'll discover that pasta substitutions aren't about limitation—they're about expansion. Each alternative opens up new flavor combinations, texture experiences, and nutritional benefits that enhance rather than restrict your cooking repertoire. Welcome to a world where pasta night becomes not just possible, but genuinely exciting again.

Vegetable-Based Noodles: Nature's Pasta Perfection

Zucchini Noodles (Zoodles) Glycemic Impact: Virtually zero | Prep Time: 5 minutes | Best Uses: Light sauces, cold salads

Zucchini noodles have revolutionized low-carb eating, and for good reason. A single medium zucchini yields about 2 cups of noodles containing only 4 grams of carbohydrates and providing excellent hydration, potassium, and vitamin C. The key to perfect zoodles lies in proper preparation and timing.

Yellow Squash and Pattypan Alternatives Glycemic Impact: Virtually zero | Prep Time: 5 minutes | Best Uses: Heartier sauces, casseroles

Yellow squash creates slightly firmer noodles than zucchini with a subtly sweeter flavor that pairs beautifully with Italian herbs and garlic. Pattypan squash, when large enough to spiralize, offers an even more substantial texture that holds up well to chunky meat sauces and baked casserole preparations.

Preparation Secrets: Always salt spiralized zucchini and let drain for 15-20 minutes before cooking. This removes excess moisture that would otherwise water down your sauce. Pat dry thoroughly before adding to hot pans. For raw applications like cold salads, the salting step is even more critical.

Cooking Techniques: Zoodles need only 1-2 minutes of cooking time. Sauté quickly in a hot pan with minimal oil, or toss with hot sauce and let residual heat warm them through. Overcooking turns them mushy and releases excess water that dilutes flavors.

Best Pairings: Light olive oil-based sauces, pesto, marinara (drained of excess liquid), carbonara-style preparations with eggs and cheese, and Asian-inspired stir-fries work beautifully with zucchini noodles.

Hearts of Palm: The Elegant Alternative

Glycemic Impact: Virtually zero | Best Uses: Elegant presentations, seafood dishes

Hearts of palm represent one of the most successful pasta substitutes for those seeking authentic texture and appearance. Available fresh in some specialty markets or canned/jarred in most grocery stores, hearts of palm naturally separate into linguine-like strands when gently pulled apart with a fork.

Nutritional Benefits: Each serving provides only 4 grams of carbohydrates while delivering potassium, vitamin B6, and a satisfying, slightly tangy flavor that enhances rather than competes with pasta sauces.

Preparation Techniques: Fresh hearts of palm should be blanched for 30 seconds in salted water, then shocked in ice water to maintain their crisp texture. Canned or jarred varieties need only to be drained and gently separated into strands. Never overcook hearts of palm, as they become mushy quickly.

Sauce Compatibility: The subtle flavor and delicate texture of hearts of palm work beautifully with seafood-based sauces, light cream sauces, olive oil and herb preparations, and fresh tomato combinations. Avoid overly heavy or chunky sauces that can overwhelm the delicate strands.

Storage and Shopping: Fresh hearts of palm keep for 3-4 days refrigerated and should feel firm when squeezed gently. Canned varieties should be transferred to glass containers after opening and used within 3 days. Look for brands that use minimal additives and avoid those with added sugars.

Rice-Based Options: Familiar Comfort

Brown Rice Pasta Glycemic Impact: Moderate | Best Uses: Traditional Italian dishes, family-friendly meals

Brown rice pasta offers the most familiar texture and appearance to traditional wheat pasta, making it an excellent choice for family meals where you want to minimize the perception of "special diet" food. The whole grain brown rice provides fiber and B-vitamins while maintaining a relatively moderate impact on blood sugar.

Wild Rice and Rice Blend Pastas Glycemic Impact: Moderate | Best Uses: Rustic, hearty preparations

Pastas made from wild rice or rice blends offer more complex flavors and additional nutrients compared to plain white rice pasta. The nuttier taste and slightly chewier texture work particularly well with mushroom-based sauces and fall vegetable combinations.

Cooking Success: Brown rice pasta can become gummy if overcooked, so watch timing carefully and rinse with cold water immediately after draining to stop the cooking process. Adding a tablespoon of olive oil to the cooking water can help prevent sticking.

Personal Preferences: Everyone's diabetes is different, and you may find that some types of pasta hit your blood sugar harder than others. Personally, rice based pastas are tough for me to take, but are easier on others. Please do your own research and ensure that you are choosing the pasta type that works best for your body.

Shirataki Noodles: The Zero-Impact Wonder

Glycemic Impact: Zero | Best Uses: Asian dishes, large portion meals
Made from the root of the konjac plant, shirataki noodles contain virtually no digestible carbohydrates, making them completely neutral for blood sugar management. This makes them particularly valuable for those times when you want a generous portion of "pasta" without any metabolic concerns.

Understanding the Texture: Shirataki noodles have a unique, slightly chewy texture that's quite different from wheat pasta. Rather than trying to replicate traditional pasta dishes exactly, embrace their distinctive quality and use them in applications where their texture enhances the dish.

Flavor Absorption: Shirataki noodles readily absorb the flavors of whatever sauce or broth they're cooked in, making them excellent vehicles for bold, well-seasoned preparations. They work particularly well in Asian-inspired dishes with ginger, garlic, soy sauce, and chili elements.

Preparation Essentials: Always rinse shirataki noodles thoroughly under cold running water for 2-3 minutes to remove the natural odor from their packaging liquid. Some people prefer to dry-roast them in a hot pan for 2-3 minutes after rinsing to improve texture, though this step isn't necessary for everyone.

Varieties and Applications: Angel hair shirataki works well in soups and light sauces, while fettuccine-width varieties can handle heartier preparations. The rice-shaped shirataki makes an excellent substitute for risotto or pilaf-style dishes.

Ancient Grain Alternatives

Quinoa Pasta Glycemic Impact: Low to moderate | Best Uses: Protein-focused meals, gluten-free family dining

Quinoa pasta provides complete protein and has a slightly nutty flavor that complements both traditional Italian sauces and more adventurous flavor combinations. The protein content helps moderate blood sugar response while providing excellent satiety.

Corn Pasta Glycemic Impact: Moderate to high | Best Uses: Mexican-inspired dishes, occasional treats

While corn pasta has a higher glycemic impact than other alternatives, it can be enjoyed occasionally when paired with plenty of protein, healthy fats, and non-starchy vegetables. The corn flavor works particularly well with southwestern and Mexican-inspired preparations.

Preparation

When preparing quinoa or corn pasta, the key to success lies in gentle handling and precise timing. Always cook in plenty of well-salted water (or low-sodium broth for extra flavor), stirring frequently during the first few minutes to prevent sticking. Both quinoa and corn pastas cook quickly and can become mushy if overdone, so remove them just shy of al dente—usually a minute earlier than package directions suggest. Avoid rapid boiling, which can cause corn pasta to split, and instead maintain a gentle simmer.

Once cooked, drain carefully (a slotted spoon works best for fragile shapes) and rinse briefly under warm water to wash away excess starch. Toss immediately with olive oil or sauce to maintain separation and enhance texture. These pastas pair beautifully with light, fresh sauces featuring olive oil, lemon, and herbs, which complement their subtle sweetness and naturally nutty flavor.

Legume-Based Pastas: Protein Powerhouses

Chickpea Pasta Glycemic Impact: Low to moderate | Best Uses: Traditional pasta dishes, meal prep

Chickpea pasta represents perhaps the closest alternative to traditional wheat pasta in terms of texture, appearance, and cooking behavior. Made entirely from ground chickpeas, it provides significantly more protein and fiber than wheat pasta while maintaining familiar cooking methods.

Nutritional Advantages: A 2-ounce serving provides approximately 11 grams of protein and 5 grams of fiber, compared to wheat pasta's 7 grams of protein and 2 grams of fiber. This protein and fiber combination helps moderate blood sugar response while providing genuine satiety.

Cooking Techniques: Chickpea pasta cooks similarly to wheat pasta but requires careful attention to prevent overcooking, which can result in mushiness. Start checking for doneness 1-2 minutes before the package directions suggest, as cooking times can vary between brands.

Sauce Compatibility: The slightly nutty flavor of chickpea pasta pairs beautifully with Mediterranean-inspired sauces, pesto, tomato-based preparations, and cream sauces. It's substantial enough to handle chunky meat sauces and vegetable combinations.

Legume-Based Pastas: Protein Powerhouses

Black Bean Pasta Glycemic Impact: Low | Prep Time: 8-10 minutes | Best Uses: Mexican-inspired dishes, bold flavor combinations

Black bean pasta offers one of the highest protein contents among legume pastas, with some brands providing up to 25 grams of protein per serving. The distinctive black color and earthy flavor work particularly well with southwestern and Mexican-inspired flavor profiles.

Lentil Pasta Glycemic Impact: Low | Best Uses: Hearty sauces, fall/winter dishes

Available in red lentil, green lentil, and black lentil varieties, lentil pastas offer distinct flavors and colors that can enhance the visual appeal of your dishes. Red lentil pasta tends to be mildest in flavor and closest to traditional pasta in appearance.

Cooking Characteristics: Lentil pasta cooks more quickly than wheat pasta and can become mushy if overcooked. Red lentil varieties typically need 6-7 minutes, while green and black lentil pastas may require 8-9 minutes. Always test for doneness frequently.

Nutritional Profile: Lentil pasta provides 13-15 grams of protein per serving along with significant amounts of folate, iron, and potassium. The high fiber content (typically 6-8 grams per serving) helps slow glucose absorption.

Cooking Techniques and Tips for Perfect Results

Sauce Pairing Strategy: Match delicate pasta alternatives like hearts of palm and shirataki with lighter sauces, while using heartier legume pastas for robust, chunky preparations. Consider the absorption properties of each alternative when choosing sauce consistency.

Texture Preservation: Most pasta alternatives benefit from slightly undercooking rather than overcooking. They continue to soften when mixed with hot sauce, so aim for a texture that's slightly firmer than your final desired result.

Storage and Meal Prep: Vegetable noodles are best prepared fresh, while legume pastas can be batch-cooked and stored for up to 4 days. Shirataki noodles store well after cooking and actually improve in texture when reheated.

Portion Considerations: Because many pasta alternatives are lower in calories than wheat pasta, you may need larger volumes to achieve satisfaction. However, the higher protein and fiber content of legume pastas often makes standard portions more filling than expected.

Family Acceptance: Introduce pasta alternatives gradually, starting with the closest textures to traditional pasta (chickpea, brown rice) before exploring more adventurous options. Serve familiar sauces with new pasta types to ease the transition.

The journey of discovering pasta alternatives is one of the most rewarding aspects of celiabetic cooking. Each option offers unique benefits and possibilities, transforming what might seem like a dietary restriction into an opportunity for culinary exploration and improved nutrition. With this comprehensive guide as your foundation, pasta night can become not just possible, but genuinely exciting again.

CHAPTER 12

Sides That Shine

Side dishes are the quiet heroes of the table—versatile companions that can elevate any meal from ordinary to memorable. In a gluten-free, diabetes-friendly kitchen, sides are where vibrant vegetables, bold flavors, and creative techniques shine brightest. Whether it's a crisp, refreshing salad, perfectly roasted seasonal produce, or a light and flavorful sauté, these recipes prove that sides don't have to play second fiddle. They add color, texture, and balance to your plate, transforming simple proteins into satisfying, well-rounded meals that never feel restrictive.

List of Recipes

1. Honey-Glazed Rainbow Carrots
2. Crispy Smashed Potatoes with Herbs
3. Asian-Style Green Beans with Almonds
4. Maple-Dijon Roasted Brussels Sprouts
5. Mediterranean Roasted Eggplant
6. Spiced Roasted Cauliflower with Tahini
7. Roasted Cauliflower Steaks with Pepitas
8. Grilled Zucchini and Peach Skewers
9. Roasted Delicata Squash with Sage

Honey-Glazed Rainbow Carrots

Vibrant heirloom carrots glazed with honey and fresh thyme create an elegant side that's both beautiful and delicious.

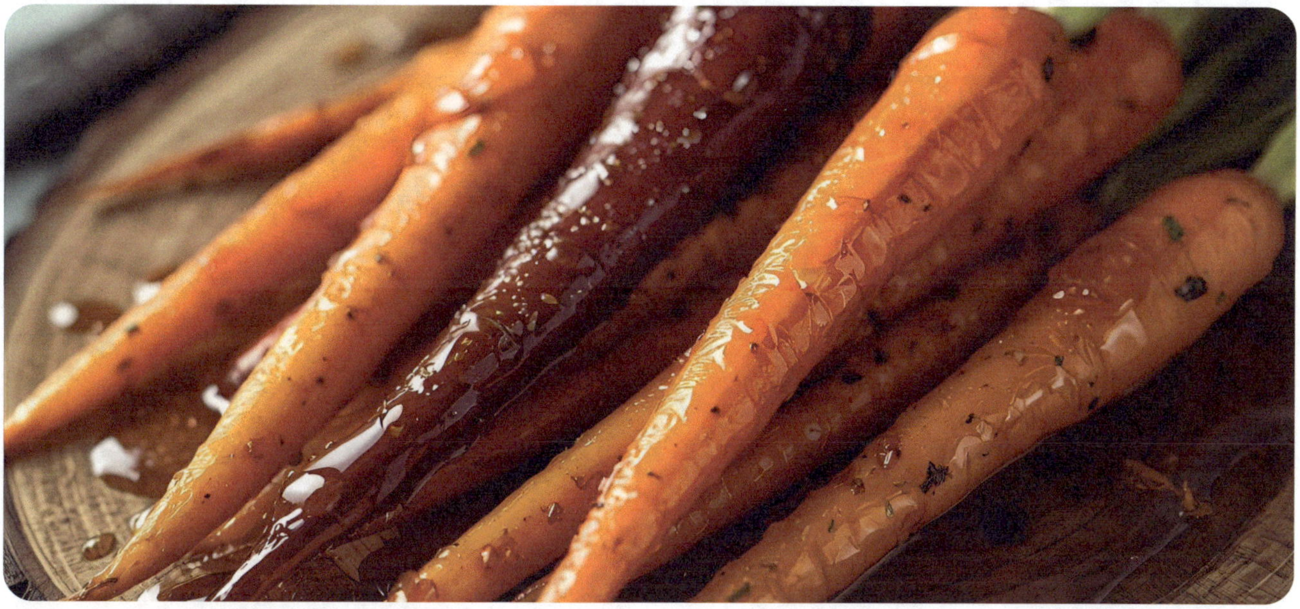

INGREDIENTS

- 2 lbs rainbow carrots (or regular carrots), peeled
- 3 tablespoons olive oil
- 3 tablespoons honey
- 2 tablespoons fresh thyme leaves
- 1 tablespoon balsamic vinegar
- 3 cloves garlic, minced
- 1/2 teaspoon salt
- 1/4 teaspoon black pepper
- 1/4 teaspoon red pepper flakes
- 2 tablespoons fresh parsley, chopped
- 2 tablespoons toasted pine nuts

6 | 10 minutes | 20 minutes

DIRECTIONS

1. Preheat oven to 425°F (220°C).
2. Toss carrots with olive oil, salt, and pepper on large rimmed baking sheet.
3. Roast 15 minutes until carrots are tender-crisp.
4. Meanwhile, whisk together honey, thyme, balsamic vinegar, garlic, and red pepper flakes.
5. Drizzle honey mixture over carrots and toss to coat.
6. Roast 5 minutes more until carrots are glazed and caramelized.
7. Garnish with fresh parsley and toasted pine nuts before serving.

NUTRITION

Per serving: 135 calories, 2g protein, 18g carbohydrates, 7g fat, 4g fiber

STORAGE

Best served immediately, but keeps for up to 2 days refrigerated. Reheat in 350°F oven.

Crispy Smashed Potatoes with Herbs

Servings	Prep time	Cook time
8	15 minutes	45 minutes

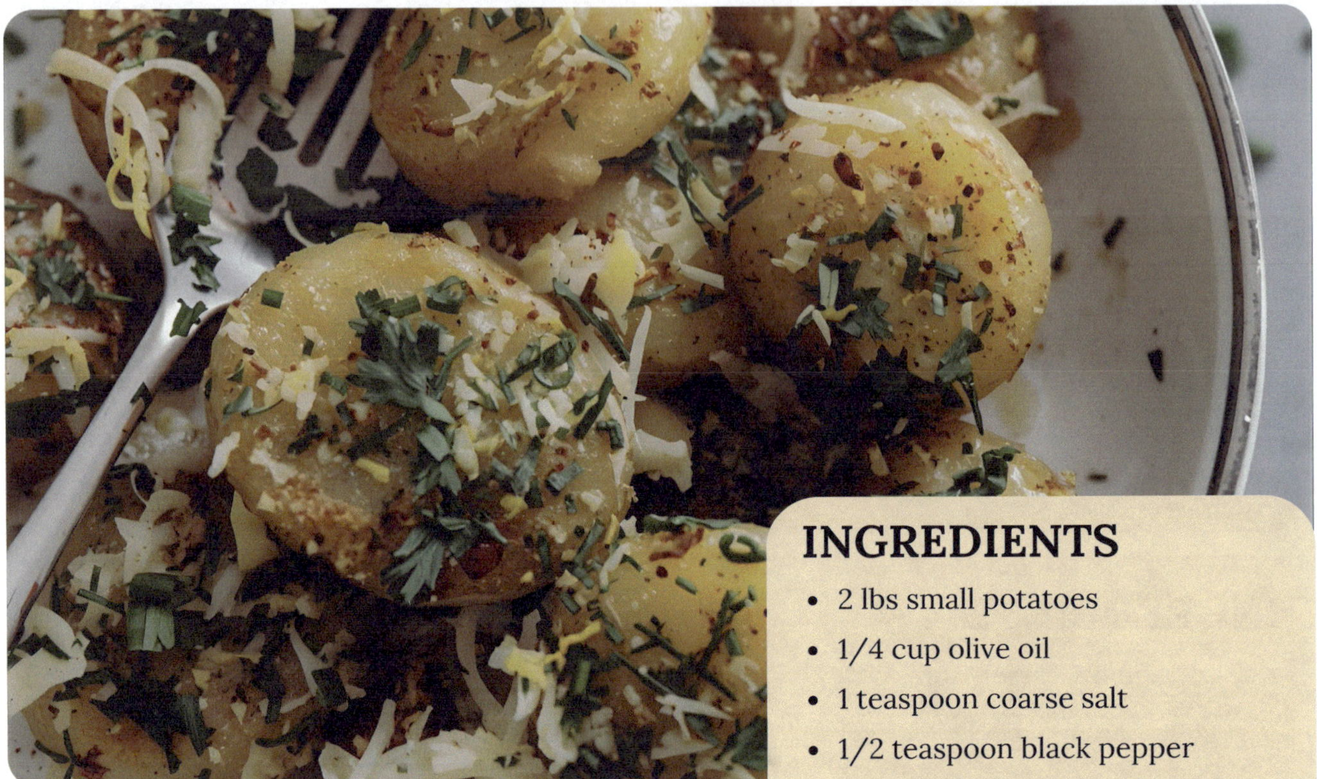

Tender inside, crispy outside potatoes with a fragrant herb topping that makes them irresistible.

INGREDIENTS

- 2 lbs small potatoes
- 1/4 cup olive oil
- 1 teaspoon coarse salt
- 1/2 teaspoon black pepper
- 1/4 cup fresh chives, chopped
- 2 tablespoons fresh dill, chopped
- 2 tablespoons fresh parsley, chopped
- 2 cloves garlic, minced
- 2 tablespoons lemon zest
- 1/4 cup Parmesan cheese, grated (optional)

DIRECTIONS

1. Preheat oven to 450°F (230°C).
2. Boil potatoes in salted water until fork-tender, about 15-20 minutes.
3. Drain potatoes and let cool slightly.
4. Place potatoes on large rimmed baking sheet. Using potato masher or fork, gently smash each potato to about 1/2-inch thickness.
5. Drizzle with olive oil and season with salt and pepper.
6. Roast 25-30 minutes until edges are golden and crispy.
7. Meanwhile, combine chives, dill, parsley, garlic, and lemon zest.
8. Top hot potatoes with herb mixture and Parmesan if using.

NUTRITION

Per serving: 145 calories, 3g protein, 22g carbohydrates, 7g fat, 3g fiber

STORAGE

Can be boiled and smashed 1 day ahead. Roast just before serving.

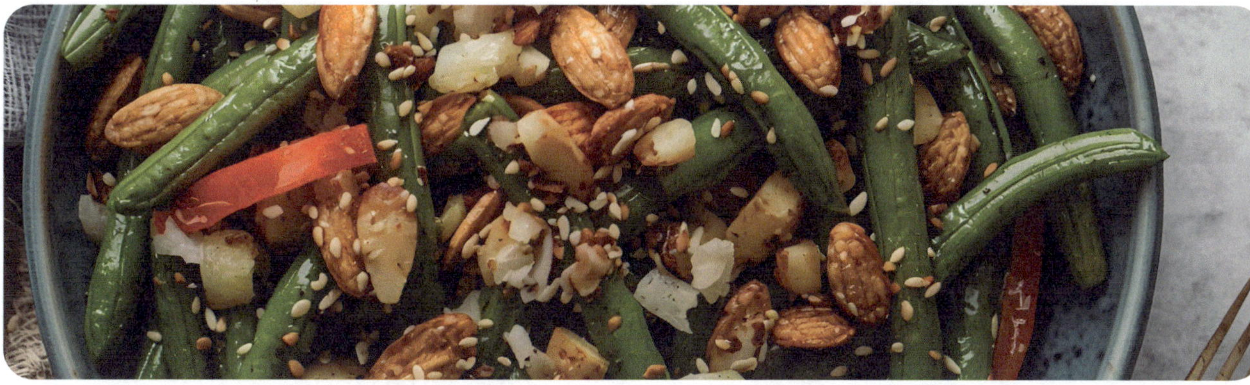

Asian-Style Green Beans with Almonds

Servings	Prep time	Cook time
6	10 minutes	8 minutes

INGREDIENTS

- 1 1/2 lbs fresh green beans, trimmed
- 2 tablespoons sesame oil
- 1/3 cup sliced almonds
- 3 cloves garlic, minced
- 1 tablespoon fresh ginger, minced
- 2 tablespoons low-sodium soy sauce (gluten-free)
- 1 tablespoon rice vinegar
- 1 teaspoon honey
- 1/4 teaspoon red pepper flakes
- 2 green onions, sliced
- 1 tablespoon sesame seeds

Crisp-tender green beans with ginger, garlic, and toasted almonds for a fresh take on a classic vegetable.

DIRECTIONS

1. Blanch green beans in boiling salted water for 3 minutes until bright green and crisp-tender. Drain and set aside.
2. Heat sesame oil in large skillet or wok over medium-high heat.
3. Add sliced almonds and toast until golden, about 2 minutes. Remove and set aside.
4. Add garlic and ginger to same pan, cooking 30 seconds until fragrant.
5. Add green beans and stir-fry 2 minutes.
6. In small bowl, whisk together soy sauce, rice vinegar, honey, and red pepper flakes.
7. Add sauce to green beans and toss to coat.
8. Remove from heat and top with toasted almonds, green onions, and sesame seeds.

NUTRITION

Per serving: 105 calories, 4g protein, 9g carbohydrates, 7g fat, 4g fiber

STORAGE

Best served immediately for optimal texture.

Maple-Dijon Roasted Brussels Sprouts

Brussels sprouts roasted until caramelized with a sweet-tangy glaze that converts even the most skeptical diners.

8	15 minutes	25 minutes

INGREDIENTS

- 2 lbs Brussels sprouts, trimmed and halved
- 1/4 cup olive oil
- 3 tablespoons sugar-free maple syrup
- 2 tablespoons Dijon mustard
- 2 tablespoons apple cider vinegar
- 4 slices bacon, chopped (optional)
- 1/3 cup dried cranberries
- 1/4 cup toasted pecans, chopped
- Salt and black pepper to taste

DIRECTIONS

1. Preheat oven to 425°F (220°C).
2. If using bacon, cook in large oven-safe skillet until crispy. Remove and set aside, leaving fat in pan.
3. Toss Brussels sprouts with olive oil (or use bacon fat), salt, and pepper.
4. Arrange cut-side down on large rimmed baking sheet or in the skillet.
5. Roast 20 minutes until caramelized and tender.
6. Meanwhile, whisk together maple syrup, Dijon mustard, and apple cider vinegar.
7. Drizzle glaze over Brussels sprouts and roast 5 minutes more.
8. Top with bacon (if using), cranberries, and toasted pecans before serving.

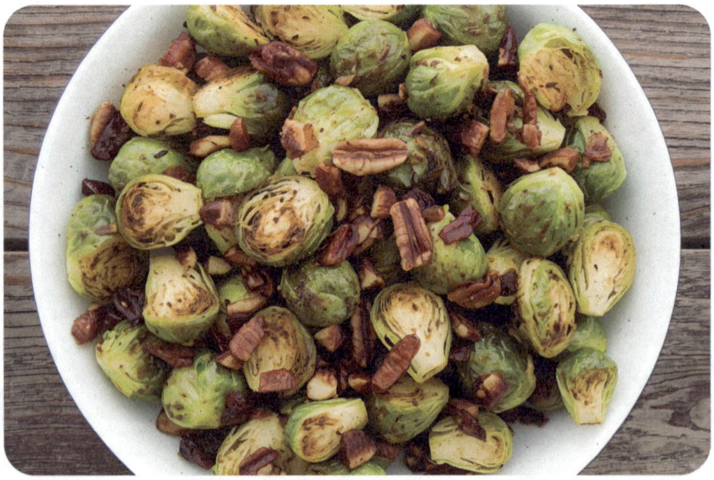

NUTRITION

Per serving: 145 calories, 5g protein, 16g carbohydrates, 8g fat, 5g fiber

STORAGE

Can be prepped 1 day ahead. Roast just before serving.

Mediterranean Roasted Eggplant

Servings	Prep time	Cook time
6	20 minutes	30 minutes

Silky roasted eggplant with Mediterranean herbs and a tangy pomegranate molasses glaze.

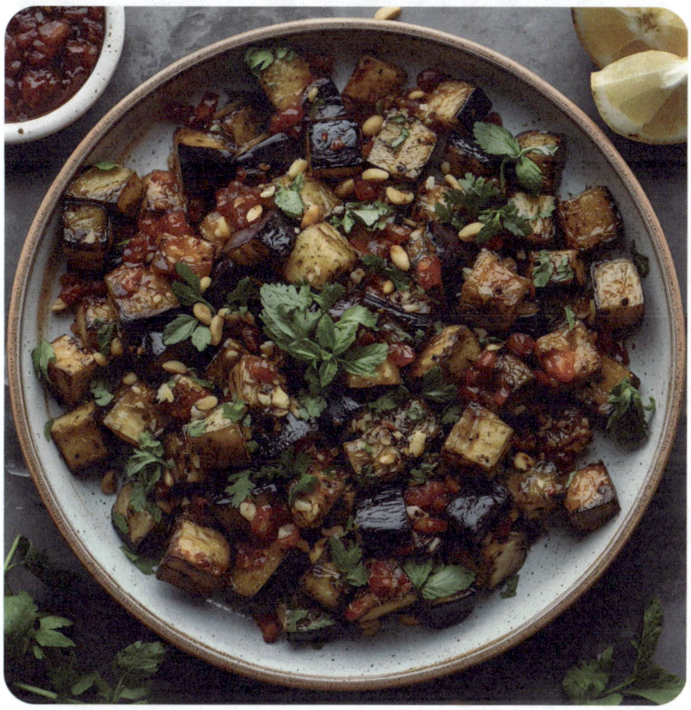

INGREDIENTS

- 2 large eggplants, cut into 1-inch cubes
- 1/4 cup olive oil
- 1 large onion, diced
- 4 cloves garlic, minced
- 1 can (14 oz) diced tomatoes, drained
- 2 tablespoons pomegranate molasses (or balsamic reduction)
- 2 teaspoons dried oregano
- 1 teaspoon ground cumin
- 1/2 cup fresh parsley, chopped
- 1/4 cup fresh mint, chopped
- 1/4 cup pine nuts, toasted
- Salt and black pepper to taste

DIRECTIONS

1. Preheat oven to 425°F (220°C).
2. Toss eggplant cubes with 3 tablespoons olive oil, salt, and pepper.
3. Spread on large rimmed baking sheet and roast 25 minutes until golden and tender.
4. Meanwhile, heat remaining olive oil in large skillet over medium heat.
5. Add onion and cook 6 minutes until softened. Add garlic and cook 1 minute.
6. Add diced tomatoes, pomegranate molasses, oregano, and cumin. Simmer 10 minutes.
7. Add roasted eggplant to skillet and toss to combine.
8. Remove from heat and stir in fresh herbs.
9. Top with toasted pine nuts before serving.

NUTRITION

Per serving: 135 calories, 4g protein, 16g carbohydrates, 8g fat, 6g fiber

STORAGE

Improves with time. Keeps for up to 3 days refrigerated. Serve at room temperature.

Spiced Roasted Cauliflower with Tahini

Middle Eastern-spiced cauliflower with a creamy tahini drizzle that transforms this humble vegetable into something extraordinary.

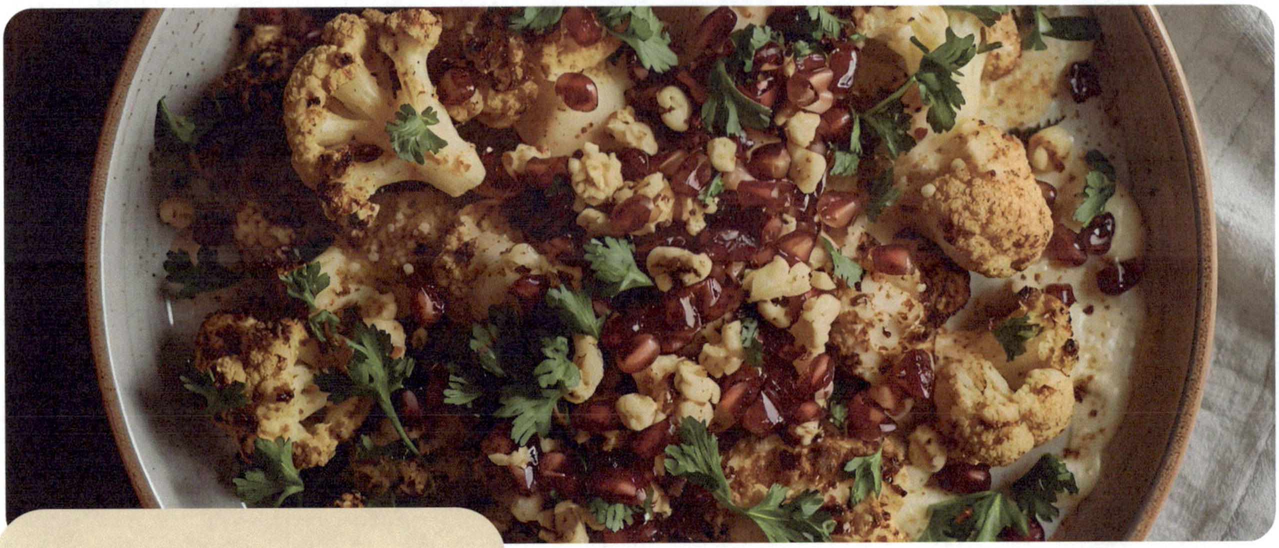

INGREDIENTS

For cauliflower:

- 1 large head cauliflower, cut into florets
- 3 tablespoons olive oil
- 1 teaspoon ground cumin
- 1 teaspoon ground coriander
- 1/2 teaspoon turmeric
- 1/2 teaspoon smoked paprika
- 1/4 teaspoon cinnamon
- 1/4 teaspoon cayenne pepper
- Salt and black pepper to taste

For tahini sauce:

- 1/4 cup tahini
- 2 tablespoons lemon juice
- 1 clove garlic, minced
- 2-3 tablespoons warm water
- Salt to taste

For garnish:

- 1/4 cup pomegranate seeds
- 2 tablespoons fresh parsley, chopped
- 2 tablespoons toasted pine nuts

6 | 15 minutes | 25 minutes

DIRECTIONS

1. Preheat oven to 425°F (220°C).
2. Toss cauliflower florets with olive oil and all spices until well coated.
3. Spread on large rimmed baking sheet and roast 20-25 minutes until golden and tender.
4. **Make tahini sauce:** Whisk together tahini, lemon juice, garlic, and salt. Add warm water gradually until smooth and pourable.
5. Arrange roasted cauliflower on serving platter and drizzle with tahini sauce.
6. Garnish with pomegranate seeds, parsley, and pine nuts.

NUTRITION

Per serving: 145 calories, 6g protein, 10g carbohydrates, 11g fat, 4g fiber

STORAGE

Cauliflower can be roasted 1 day ahead. Reheat and add fresh garnishes

Roasted Cauliflower Steaks with Turmeric & Pepitas

INGREDIENTS

- 1 large head cauliflower
- 3 tbsp olive oil
- 1 tsp ground turmeric
- ½ tsp garlic powder
- ¼ tsp smoked paprika
- ½ tsp salt
- ¼ tsp black pepper
- ¼ cup raw pepitas (pumpkin seeds)
- 2 tbsp chopped fresh cilantro
- 1 tbsp lemon zest
- 2 tbsp crumbled feta cheese (optional)

NUTRITION

Per serving: 160 calories, 7g protein, 11g carbohydrates, 11g fat, 5g fiber

STORAGE

Best served immediately, but leftovers can be refrigerated for 2–3 days; reheat gently.

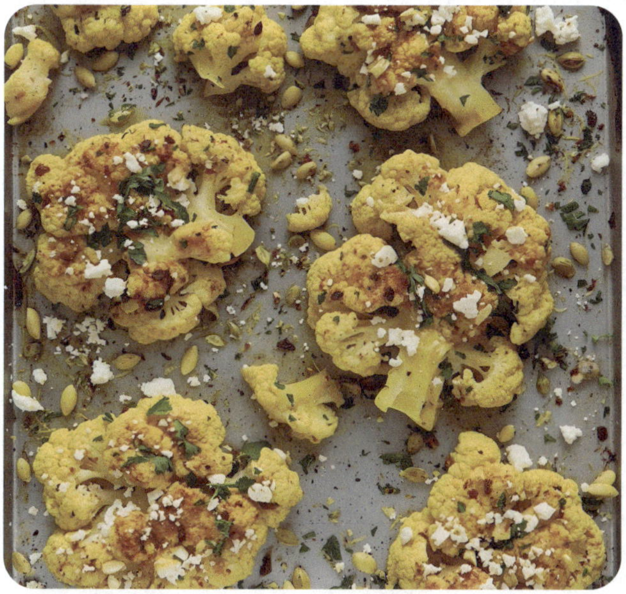

Servings	Prep time	Cook time
4	10 minutes	30 minutes

Golden roasted cauliflower "steaks" topped with crunchy pepitas, fresh herbs, and a hint of lemon zest.

DIRECTIONS

1. Preheat oven to 425°F (220°C).
2. Slice cauliflower into 1-inch "steaks" (reserve florets for another use).
3. In a small bowl, whisk olive oil, turmeric, garlic powder, paprika, salt, and pepper.
4. Brush both sides of cauliflower steaks with oil mixture. Place on a baking sheet.
5. Roast 20 minutes, carefully flip, and roast 10–15 minutes more until golden and tender.
6. Meanwhile, toast pepitas in a dry skillet until lightly golden and fragrant, then set aside.
7. Top roasted cauliflower steaks with toasted pepitas, cilantro, lemon zest, and feta, if using.
8. Serve warm.

4 | 10 minutes | 6 minutes

Grilled Zucchini & Peach Skewers

Sweet peaches and smoky zucchini skewered, grilled, and finished with balsamic glaze.

INGREDIENTS

- 2 medium zucchini, sliced into ½-inch rounds
- 2 ripe peaches, pitted and cut into wedges
- 2 tbsp olive oil
- 1 tbsp balsamic glaze
- ½ tsp sea salt
- ½ tsp black pepper
- ¼ cup crumbled goat cheese (optional)
- 2 tbsp fresh basil, chopped

DIRECTIONS

1. Preheat grill or grill pan to medium-high.
2. Toss zucchini and peach wedges with olive oil, salt, and pepper.
3. Thread zucchini and peaches alternately onto skewers.
4. Grill 2–3 minutes per side until zucchini softens and grill marks appear.
5. Drizzle with balsamic glaze, sprinkle with goat cheese and fresh basil, and serve immediately.

NUTRITION

Per serving: 110 calories, 2g protein, 10g carbohydrates, 7g fat, 2g fiber

STORAGE

Best served immediately.

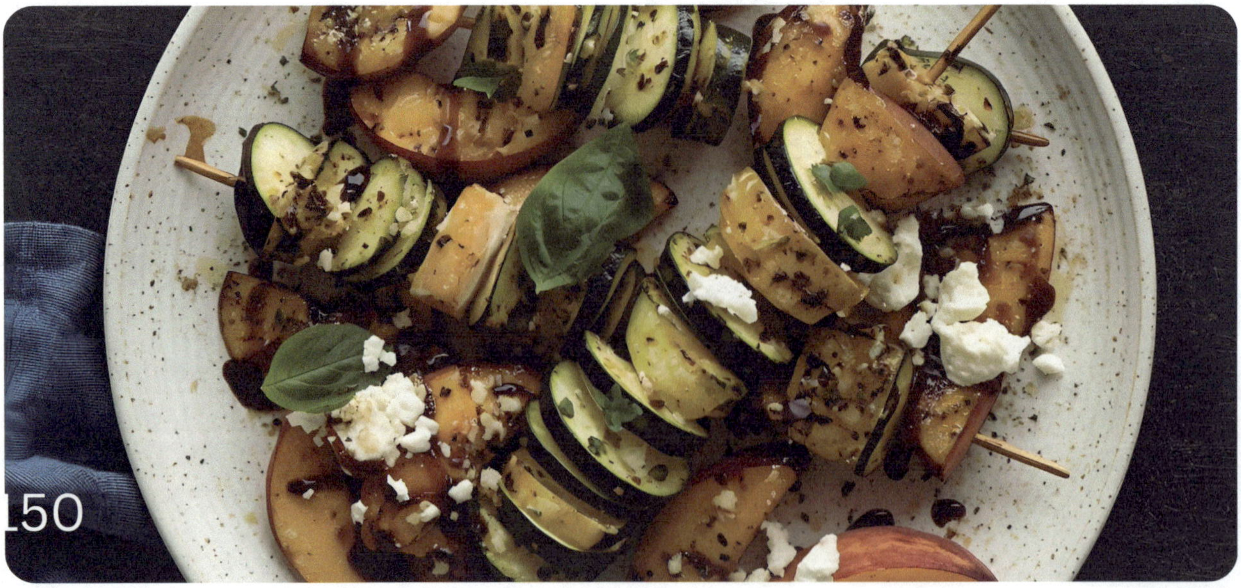

Roasted Delicata Squash with Sage

Servings	Prep time	Cook time
8	10 minutes	30 minutes

Tender roasted delicata squash with earthy sage, crunchy pepitas, and tangy vinegar.

INGREDIENTS

- 2 small delicata squash, halved lengthwise, seeded, and sliced into ½-inch half-moons
- 2 tbsp olive oil
- ½ tsp salt
- ½ tsp black pepper
- 1 tsp dried sage
- 2 tbsp pepitas (pumpkin seeds)
- 2 tbsp crumbled feta cheese (optional)
- 1 tbsp apple cider vinegar

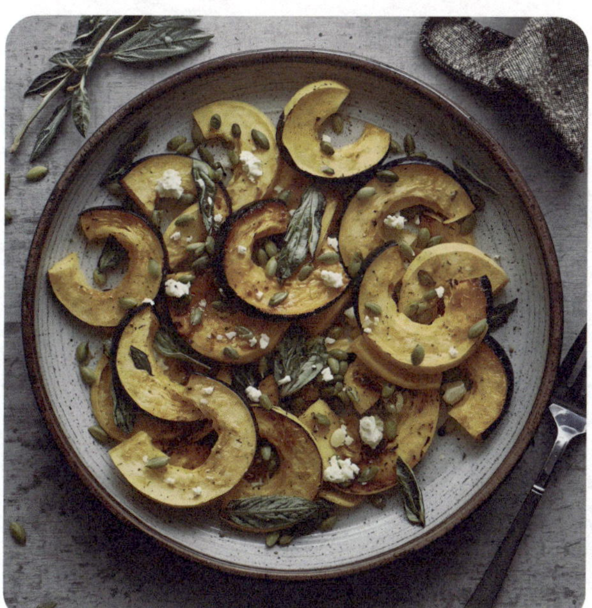

DIRECTIONS

1. Preheat oven to 400°F (200°C).
2. Toss squash with olive oil, salt, pepper, and sage. Roast on a baking sheet for 25–30 minutes until golden and tender.
3. In a dry pan, toast pepitas until fragrant, then toss with roasted squash.
4. Sprinkle with feta if using and drizzle with apple cider vinegar before serving.

NUTRITION

Per serving: 100 calories, 2g protein, 9g carbohydrates, 7g fat, 2g fiber

STORAGE

Keeps for 3 days refrigerated; reheat gently.

TIPS FOR PERFECT VEGETABLE SIDES

High Heat is Your Friend: Most vegetables benefit from high-temperature cooking (425°F+) that caramelizes surfaces while keeping interiors tender.

Don't Overcrowd: Give vegetables space to roast properly. Use multiple pans if necessary to avoid steaming.

Season in Stages: Salt vegetables before cooking to draw out moisture, then adjust seasoning after cooking for optimal flavor.

Timing Matters: Add delicate herbs and garnishes after cooking to preserve their fresh flavors and bright colors.

Embrace Seasonal Variations: Use these recipes as templates and substitute seasonal vegetables to keep sides interesting year-round.

Texture Contrast: Combine soft roasted vegetables with crunchy nuts, seeds, or crispy garnishes for more interesting eating.

Make-Ahead Strategy: Many roasted vegetables can be prepared ahead and served at room temperature or gently reheated.

Acid Brightens Everything: A splash of citrus juice, vinegar, or other acid added at the end brightens flavors and balances richness.

Quality Olive Oil Matters: Use your best extra virgin olive oil for finishing dishes – it makes a noticeable difference.

Storage Wisdom: Most roasted vegetables keep well for 2-3 days refrigerated and often taste even better the next day as flavors meld.

Remember that vegetables are incredibly forgiving and adaptable. Use these recipes as starting points and adjust seasonings, cooking times, and garnishes based on your preferences and what's available seasonally. The goal is to make vegetables so appealing that they become the part of the meal everyone looks forward to most.

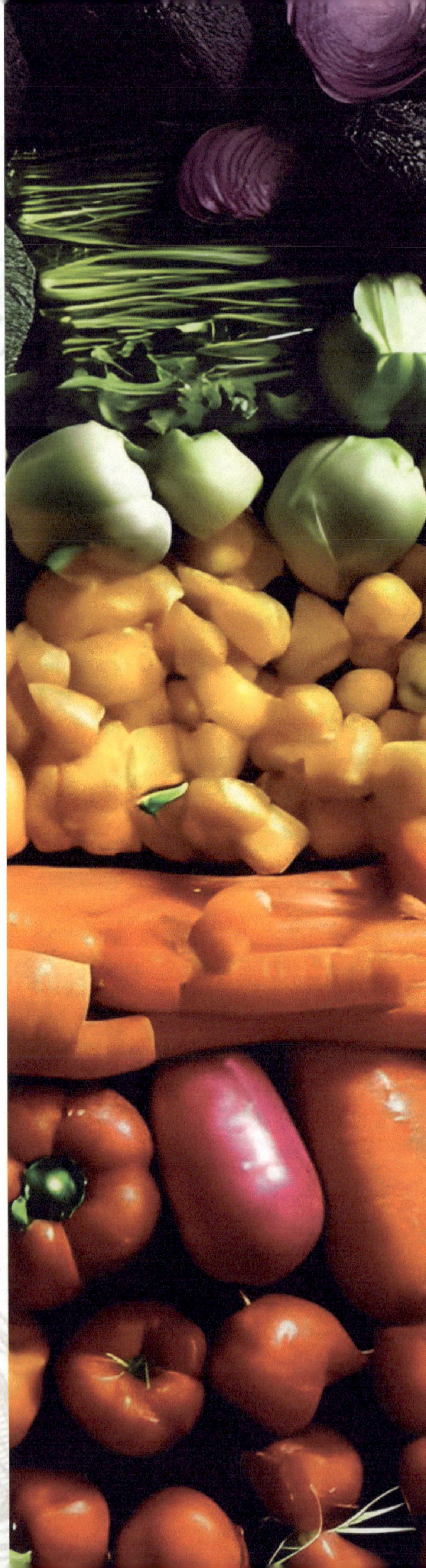

CHAPTER 13

Grain & Legume Sides

Grains and legumes form the nutritional backbone of healthy eating around the world, providing sustained energy, complete proteins, and essential nutrients that support both diabetes management and overall wellness. These humble ingredients deserve recognition as true superfoods – offering fiber that helps stabilize blood sugar, plant-based proteins that satisfy hunger, and complex carbohydrates that provide steady energy without dramatic glucose spikes.

List of Recipes

1. Smokey Chickpea and Kale Saute
2. Herbed Quinoa Pilaf
3. Mediterranean White Bean Salad
4. Coconut Rice with Cilantro and Lime
5. Spiced Lentil and Rice Pilaf
6. Cuban Black Beans and Rice
7. Brown Rice Salad with Roasted Vegetables
8. Three-Bean Chili Side

The Nutritional Power of Beans and Legumes

Legumes—including beans, lentils, chickpeas, and peas—are nutritional powerhouses offering unique advantages for people managing both celiac disease and diabetes.
Their greatest strength is fiber content, especially soluble fiber, which slows glucose absorption and promotes steadier blood sugar levels. Instead of sharp peaks and valleys from refined carbohydrates, legumes create a gentle, sustained rise in glucose. Studies show that eating legumes regularly improves blood sugar control, lowers cholesterol, and reduces cardiovascular disease risk.

Legumes provide plant-based protein paired with complex carbohydrates and fiber, creating steady energy while keeping you fuller longer. This satiety factor makes them powerful allies in weight management and appetite control, both critical for diabetes care.

Nutritionally, legumes are rich in folate, iron, potassium, and magnesium, supporting heart health, muscle function, and energy production. Many contain resistant starch (particularly when cooked and cooled) that acts as a prebiotic, nourishing beneficial gut bacteria vital for regulating metabolism and supporting immune health.

Culinarily, legumes are endlessly adaptable. Black beans add depth to soups; lentils transform into hearty stews; chickpeas shine in curries or hummus; split peas become comforting soups. Their mild flavors readily absorb seasonings, making them perfect for global cuisines. When paired with quinoa, brown rice, or wild rice, legumes form complete proteins containing all nine essential amino acids—excellent alternatives to animal proteins.

Exploring Exotic Beans: Beyond common varieties, exotic beans offer exciting flavors and textures worth discovering. Adzuki beans bring a slightly sweet, nutty taste to both savory and dessert applications. Mung beans cook quickly and work beautifully in Asian-inspired dishes or sprouted for salads. Fava beans (broad beans) provide a buttery, earthy flavor perfect for Mediterranean dishes, while tepary beans—a drought-resistant heirloom variety—offer exceptional fiber content and a rich, complex taste. Cranberry beans (borlotti) feature a creamy texture and chestnut-like flavor that elevates Italian soups and stews. These varieties often appear in specialty stores or international markets and can transform familiar recipes into culinary adventures while delivering the same blood sugar benefits as their more common cousins.

Legumes aren't just another carbohydrate—they're a foundation for balanced eating that supports blood sugar stability, digestive health, and overall wellness.

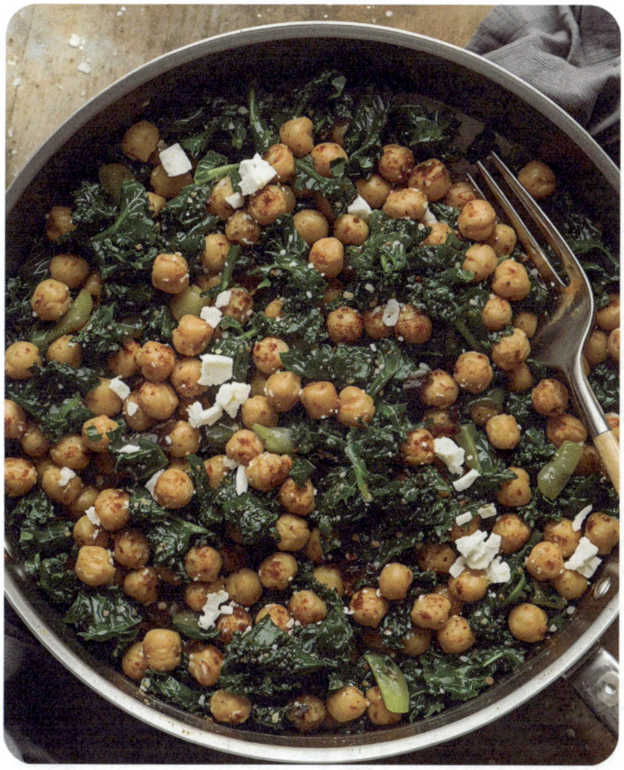

Smoky Chickpea & Kale Sauté

Hearty chickpeas and kale sautéed with smoky spices and brightened with lemon.

Servings	Prep time	Cook time
6	10 minutes	10 minutes

NUTRITION

Per serving: 185 calories, 8g protein, 20g carbohydrates, 9g fat, 7g fiber

STORAGE

Keeps for 3 days refrigerated; best reheated gently.

INGREDIENTS

- 2 cans (15 oz each) chickpeas, drained and rinsed
- 1 bunch kale, stems removed, chopped
- 3 tbsp olive oil
- 2 cloves garlic, minced
- 1 tsp smoked paprika
- ½ tsp ground cumin
- ½ tsp salt
- ¼ tsp crushed red pepper flakes
- 2 tbsp lemon juice
- 2 tbsp crumbled goat cheese (optional)

DIRECTIONS

1. Heat olive oil in a large skillet over medium heat.
2. Add garlic and sauté 1 minute until fragrant.
3. Add kale and sauté 3–4 minutes until wilted.
4. Add chickpeas, smoked paprika, cumin, salt, and red pepper flakes; cook 5 minutes, stirring occasionally.
5. Remove from heat, stir in lemon juice, and sprinkle with goat cheese if using.

Herbed Quinoa Pilaf

Servings	Prep time	Cook time
8	15 minutes	25 minutes

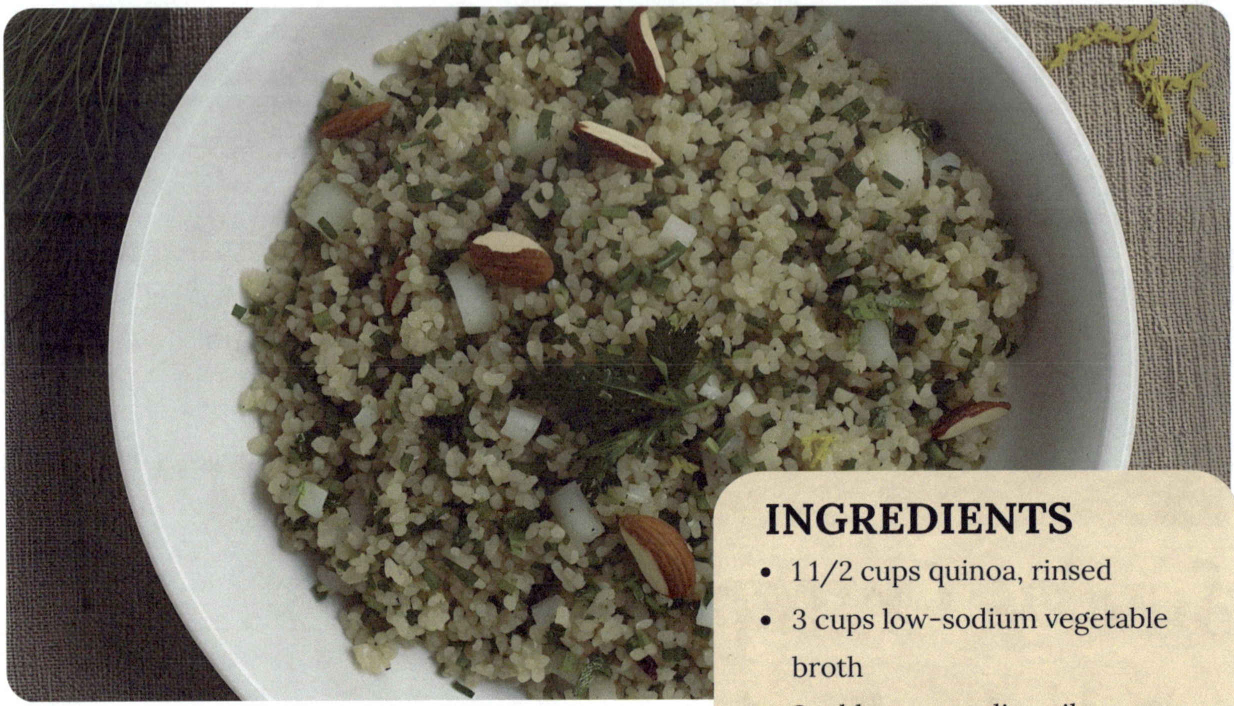

A fragrant, fluffy quinoa pilaf with fresh herbs and toasted almonds that pairs beautifully with grilled proteins.

INGREDIENTS

- 1 1/2 cups quinoa, rinsed
- 3 cups low-sodium vegetable broth
- 2 tablespoons olive oil
- 1 medium onion, finely diced
- 2 cloves garlic, minced
- 1/4 cup fresh parsley, chopped
- 2 tablespoons fresh mint, chopped
- 2 tablespoons fresh dill, chopped
- 1/3 cup toasted sliced almonds
- 2 tablespoons lemon juice
- 1 tablespoon lemon zest
- Salt and black pepper to taste

DIRECTIONS

1. Heat olive oil in large saucepan over medium heat.
2. Add onion and cook 5 minutes until softened and translucent.
3. Add garlic and cook 1 minute until fragrant.
4. Add quinoa and stir to coat with oil. Toast 2 minutes until fragrant.
5. Add broth and bring to boil. Reduce heat to low, cover, and simmer 15 minutes.
6. Remove from heat and let stand 5 minutes. Fluff with fork.
7. Stir in fresh herbs, toasted almonds, lemon juice, and lemon zest.
8. Season with salt and pepper to taste.
9. Serve warm or at room temperature.

NUTRITION

Per serving: 185 calories, 6g protein, 28g carbohydrates, 6g fat, 3g fiber

STORAGE

Keeps for up to 4 days refrigerated. Bring to room temperature before serving.

Mediterranean White Bean Salad

Servings	Prep time	Cook time
6	15 minutes	0 minutes

A protein-rich bean salad with Mediterranean flavors that improves as it marinates.

INGREDIENTS

- 2 cans (15 oz each) cannellini beans, drained and rinsed
- 1 cucumber, diced
- 1 cup cherry tomatoes, halved
- 1/2 red onion, thinly sliced
- 1/2 cup Kalamata olives, pitted and halved
- 1/2 cup fresh parsley, chopped
- 1/4 cup fresh basil, chopped
- 1/4 cup extra virgin olive oil
- 3 tablespoons red wine vinegar
- 2 cloves garlic, minced
- 1 teaspoon dried oregano
- 1/2 teaspoon salt
- 1/4 teaspoon black pepper
- 4 oz feta cheese, crumbled

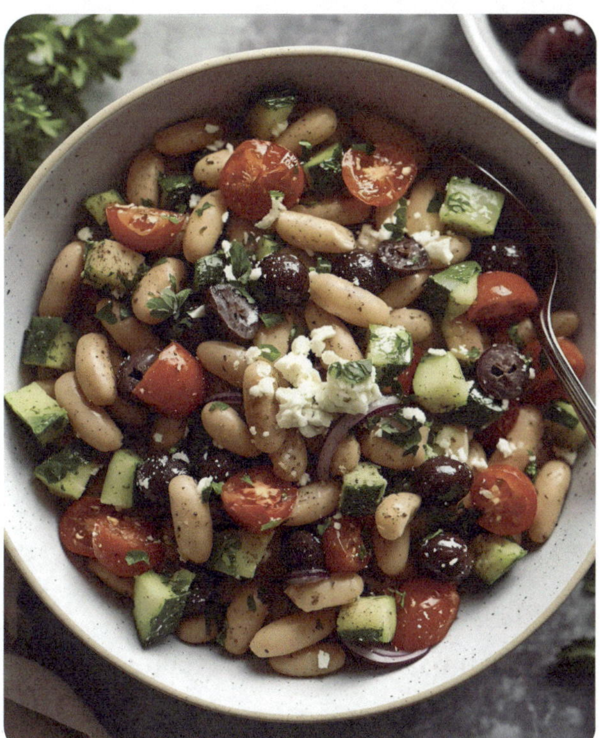

DIRECTIONS

1. In large bowl, combine beans, cucumber, tomatoes, red onion, olives, parsley, and basil.
2. In small bowl, whisk together olive oil, red wine vinegar, garlic, oregano, salt, and pepper.
3. Pour dressing over bean mixture and toss gently to combine.
4. Let marinate at room temperature 30 minutes for flavors to meld.
5. Top with crumbled feta cheese just before serving.
6. Serve at room temperature or chilled.

NUTRITION

Per serving: 265 calories, 12g protein, 26g carbohydrates, 14g fat, 8g fiber

STORAGE

Keeps for up to 3 days refrigerated. Add feta just before serving.

Coconut Rice with Cilantro and Lime

Fragrant jasmine rice cooked in coconut milk with bright herbs, perfect with Asian-inspired dishes.

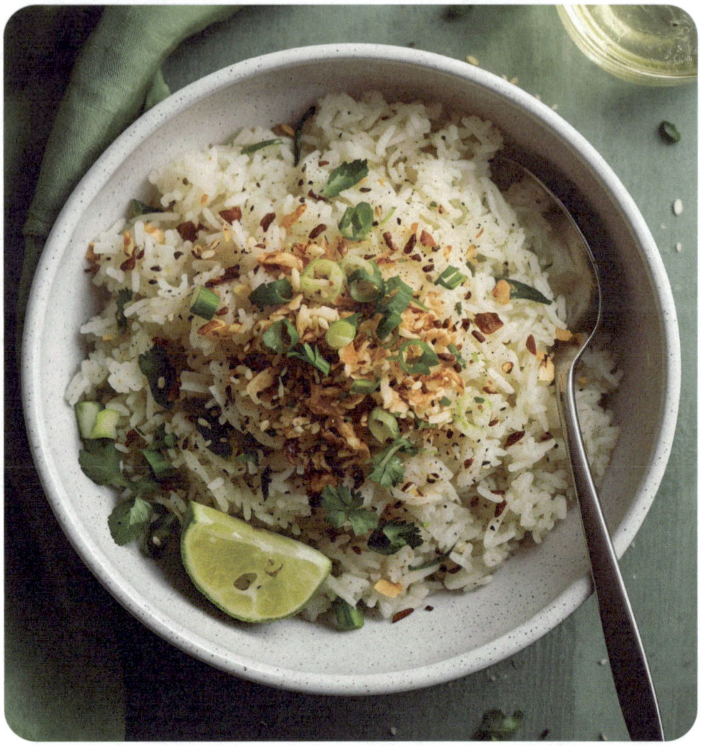

INGREDIENTS

- 1 1/2 cups jasmine rice, rinsed
- 1 can (14 oz) light coconut milk
- 1 1/4 cups water
- 1 teaspoon salt
- 2 tablespoons lime juice
- 1 tablespoon lime zest
- 1/4 cup fresh cilantro, chopped
- 2 green onions, sliced
- 2 tablespoons toasted coconut flakes
- 1 tablespoon sesame seeds

6	10 minutes	20 minutes

DIRECTION

1. In medium saucepan, combine rice, coconut milk, water, and salt.
2. Bring to boil over medium-high heat.
3. Reduce heat to low, cover, and simmer 18 minutes until liquid is absorbed.
4. Remove from heat and let stand 5 minutes.
5. Fluff rice with fork and stir in lime juice and lime zest.
6. Fold in cilantro and green onions.
7. Garnish with toasted coconut flakes and sesame seeds before serving.

NUTRITION

Per serving: 215 calories, 5g protein, 38g carbohydrates, 5g fat, 1g fiber

STORAGE

Keeps for up to 3 days refrigerated. Reheat gently in microwave or steamer.

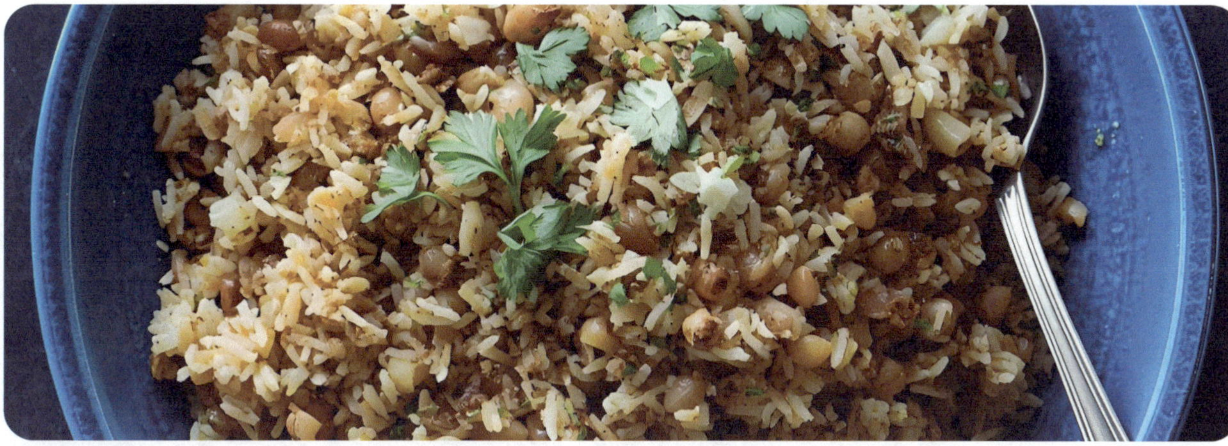

Spiced Lentil and Rice Pilaf

8 | 15 minutes | 45 minutes

INGREDIENTS

- 1 cup brown lentils, rinsed
- 1 cup long-grain white rice
- 3 large onions, thinly sliced
- 1/4 cup olive oil
- 3 1/2 cups vegetable broth
- 1 teaspoon ground cumin
- 1 teaspoon ground coriander
- 1/2 teaspoon turmeric
- 1/2 teaspoon cinnamon
- 1/4 teaspoon allspice
- 1 bay leaf
- Salt and black pepper to taste
- 1/4 cup fresh parsley, chopped
- Greek yogurt for serving (optional)

A Middle Eastern comfort food combining lentils and rice with caramelized onions and warming spices.

DIRECTIONS

1. Heat olive oil in large, heavy-bottomed pot over medium heat.
2. Add sliced onions and cook 20-25 minutes, stirring occasionally, until deep golden brown and caramelized.
3. Remove half the onions and set aside for garnish.
4. Add lentils, rice, and all spices to remaining onions in pot.
5. Stir to coat grains with spices and cook 2 minutes until fragrant.
6. Add broth and bay leaf. Bring to boil.
7. Reduce heat to low, cover, and simmer 25 minutes until lentils and rice are tender.
8. Remove bay leaf and let stand 10 minutes.
9. Fluff with fork and season with salt and pepper.
10. Garnish with reserved caramelized onions and fresh parsley.
11. Serve with Greek yogurt if desired.

NUTRITION

Per serving: 245 calories, 9g protein, 42g carbohydrates, 6g fat, 6g fiber

STORAGE

Keeps for up to 4 days refrigerated. Add water when reheating if needed.

Cuban Black Beans and Rice

A satisfying Cuban-inspired dish with perfectly seasoned black beans served over fluffy rice.

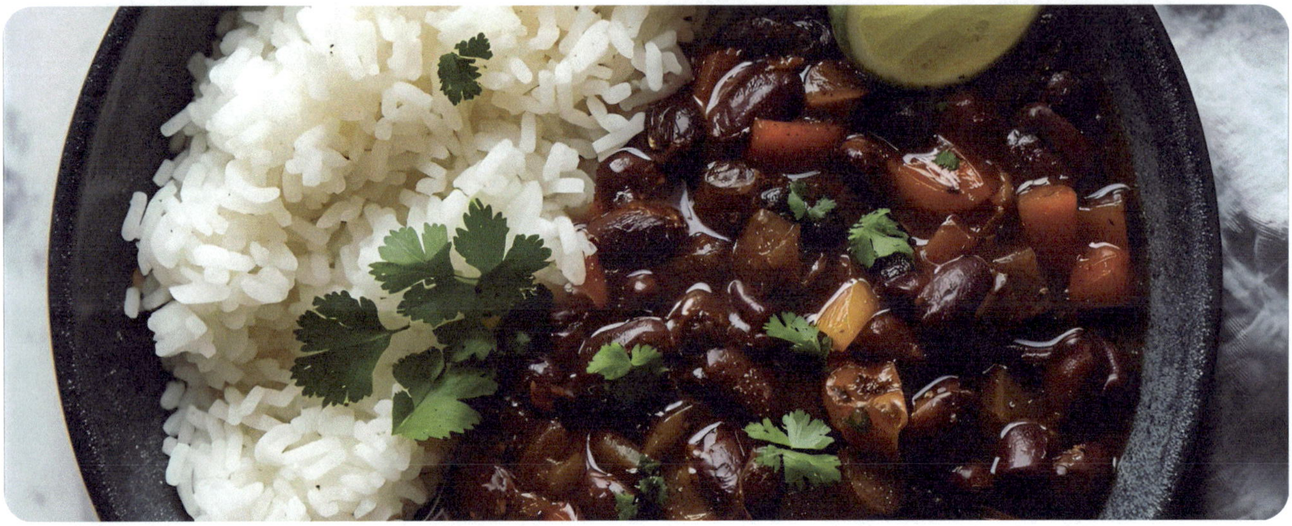

INGREDIENTS

For black beans:

- 2 cans (15 oz each) black beans, drained and rinsed
- 2 tablespoons olive oil
- 1 large onion, diced
- 1 bell pepper, diced
- 4 cloves garlic, minced
- 1 teaspoon ground cumin
- 1 teaspoon dried oregano
- 1/2 teaspoon smoked paprika
- 1 bay leaf
- 1 cup vegetable broth
- 2 tablespoons lime juice
- Salt and black pepper to taste

For rice:

- 1 1/2 cups long-grain white rice
- 3 cups water
- 1 teaspoon salt
- 1 tablespoon olive oil

For serving:

- 1/4 cup fresh cilantro, chopped
- Lime wedges
- Diced avocado (optional)

9 | 15 minutes | 35 minutes

DIRECTIONS

1. **Cook rice:** In medium saucepan, bring water, salt, and olive oil to boil. Add rice, reduce heat to low, cover, and simmer 18 minutes. Remove from heat and let stand 5 minutes.
2. **Prepare beans:** Heat olive oil in large skillet over medium heat. Add onion and bell pepper, cooking 6 minutes until softened.
3. Add garlic, cumin, oregano, and paprika. Cook 1 minute until fragrant.
4. Add black beans, bay leaf, and broth. Simmer 15 minutes until slightly thickened.
5. Remove bay leaf and stir in lime juice. Season with salt and pepper.
6. Serve beans over rice, garnished with cilantro, lime wedges, and avocado if using.

NUTRITION

Per serving: 285 calories, 10g protein, 52g carbohydrates, 5g fat, 8g fiber

STORAGE

Both components keep for up to 4 days refrigerated.

Brown Rice Salad with Roasted Vegetables

8 | 20 minutes | 45 minutes

A hearty grain salad with nutty brown rice, roasted vegetables, and fresh herbs that's naturally gluten-free.

DIRECTIONS

1. Preheat oven to 425°F (220°C).
2. Cook brown rice according to package directions (usually 45 minutes in boiling salted water). Drain and cool.
3. Toss zucchini, bell peppers, and red onion with 2 tablespoons olive oil, salt, and pepper.
4. Spread on large rimmed baking sheet and roast 20-25 minutes until tender and lightly caramelized.
5. In large bowl, combine cooled rice, roasted vegetables, sun-dried tomatoes, pine nuts, basil, and parsley.
6. In small bowl, whisk together remaining olive oil, balsamic vinegar, lemon juice, garlic, salt, and pepper.
7. Pour dressing over salad and toss to combine.
8. Let stand 30 minutes for flavors to meld.
9. Top with goat cheese if using before serving.

INGREDIENTS

- 1 1/2 cups long-grain brown rice
- 2 medium zucchini, diced
- 1 red bell pepper, diced
- 1 yellow bell pepper, diced
- 1 red onion, diced
- 1/4 cup olive oil, divided
- 1/4 cup sun-dried tomatoes, chopped
- 1/3 cup toasted pine nuts
- 1/4 cup fresh basil, chopped
- 2 tablespoons fresh parsley, chopped
- 3 tablespoons balsamic vinegar
- 2 tablespoons lemon juice
- 1 clove garlic, minced
- Salt and black pepper to taste
- 4 oz goat cheese, crumbled (optional)

NUTRITION

Per serving: 245 calories, 6g protein, 38g carbohydrates, 8g fat, 4g fiber

STORAGE

Beets can be roasted 2 days ahead. Assemble just before serving.

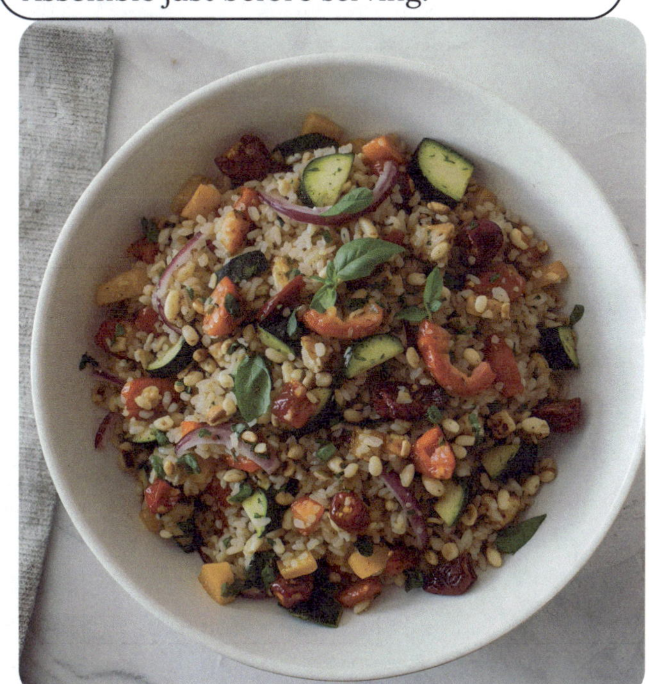

Three-Bean Chili Side

A protein-rich, meatless chili that works perfectly as a substantial side dish or light main course.

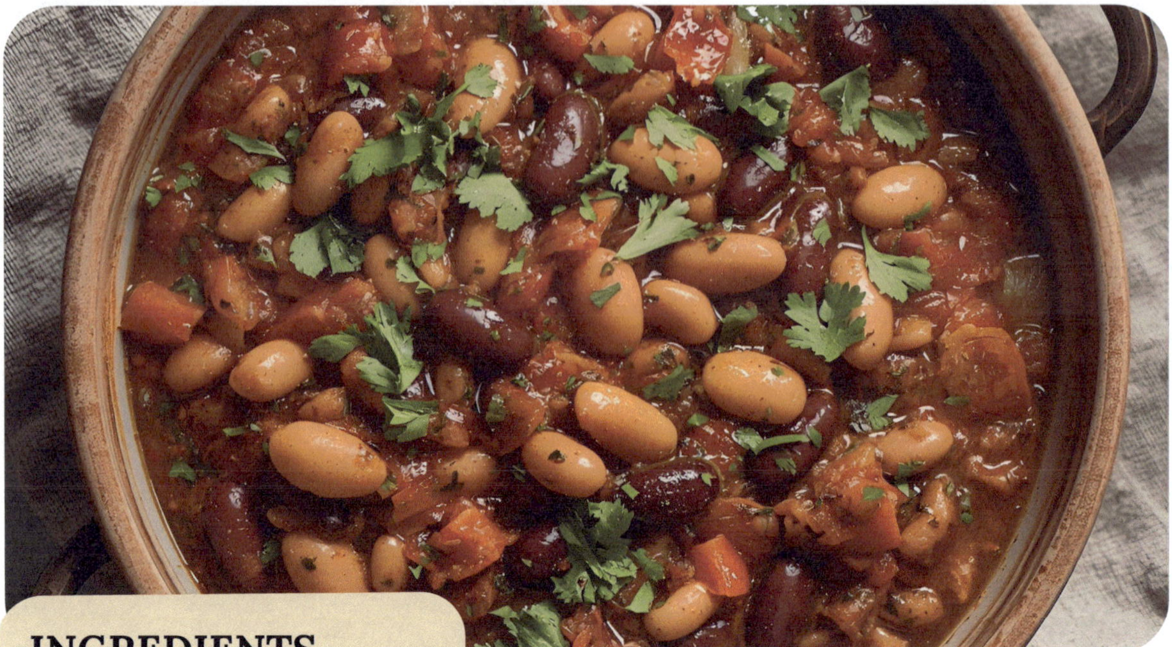

INGREDIENTS

- 1 can (15 oz) black beans, drained and rinsed
- 1 can (15 oz) pinto beans, drained and rinsed
- 1 can (15 oz) kidney beans, drained and rinsed
- 2 tablespoons olive oil
- 1 large onion, diced
- 1 bell pepper, diced
- 3 cloves garlic, minced
- 2 tablespoons chili powder
- 1 tablespoon ground cumin
- 1 teaspoon smoked paprika
- 1/2 teaspoon oregano
- 1/4 teaspoon cayenne pepper (optional)
- 1 can (28 oz) diced tomatoes
- 1 cup vegetable broth
- 1 tablespoon tomato paste
- 1 tablespoon lime juice
- Salt and black pepper to taste
- 1/4 cup fresh cilantro, chopped

10	15 minutes	15 minutes

DIRECTIONS

1. Heat olive oil in large pot over medium heat.
2. Add onion and bell pepper, cooking 6 minutes until softened.
3. Add garlic and cook 1 minute until fragrant.
4. Add chili powder, cumin, paprika, oregano, and cayenne. Cook 1 minute until fragrant.
5. Add tomato paste and cook 1 minute more.
6. Add diced tomatoes, broth, and all beans. Bring to boil.
7. Reduce heat and simmer 25 minutes until slightly thickened.
8. Stir in lime juice and season with salt and pepper.
9. Garnish with fresh cilantro before serving.

NUTRITION

Per serving: 165 calories, 9g protein, 28g carbohydrates, 3g fat, 10g fiber

STORAGE

Freezes beautifully for up to 4 months.

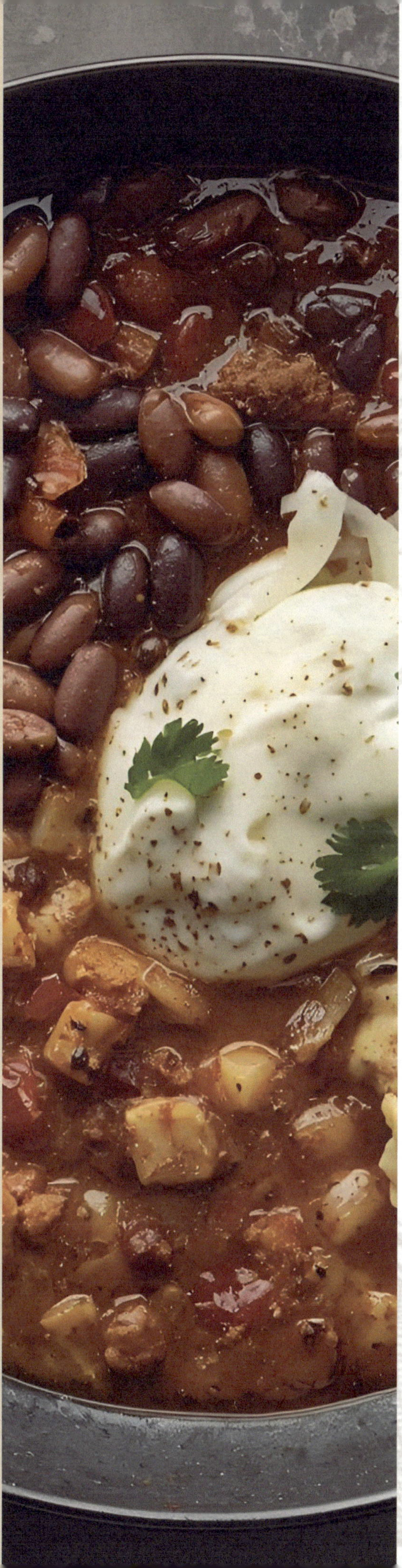

TIPS FOR ONE-PAN SUCCESS

Rinse Before Cooking: Always rinse grains and legumes in cold water until water runs clear to remove excess starch and debris.

Proper Ratios: Most grains use a 2:1 liquid-to-grain ratio, but this varies. Always check package directions for specific requirements.

Toast for Flavor: Toasting grains in oil before adding liquid enhances their nutty flavor significantly.

Season the Cooking Water: Add salt to cooking water for grains and legumes to enhance flavor from the inside out.

Don't Rush the Process: Grains and legumes need adequate cooking time to achieve proper texture. Undercooking results in hard, unpalatable grains.

Let Them Rest: After cooking, let grains rest off heat for 5-10 minutes before fluffing to ensure even texture.

Batch Cooking Benefits: Cook larger quantities and refrigerate or freeze portions for quick meal assembly throughout the week.

Soaking Advantages: While not always necessary, soaking beans and whole grains can reduce cooking time and improve digestibility.

Storage Solutions: Cooked grains and legumes keep 3-5 days refrigerated and freeze well for up to 3 months.

Flavor Layering: Build flavors by cooking grains in broth instead of water, and add aromatics like bay leaves, herbs, or spices during cooking.

Texture Preferences: Cooking times can be adjusted based on texture preferences – longer for softer, shorter for more al dente results.

Make-Ahead Advantages: Most grain and legume dishes actually improve in flavor when made ahead, making them perfect for meal prep and entertaining.

Remember that grains and legumes are incredibly versatile and forgiving. These recipes provide frameworks that can be adapted based on seasonal ingredients, personal preferences, and what you have available in your pantry

CHAPTER 14

Wholesome Sweets and Desserts

The myth that managing celiac disease and diabetes means abandoning dessert ends here. This chapter proves that when you build desserts with wholesome ingredients like almond flour, natural sweeteners, and fresh fruits, you create treats that are genuinely satisfying without the blood sugar rollercoaster or gluten-related damage. These aren't sad substitutes—they're desserts so delicious that everyone at the table will want the recipe, regardless of dietary restrictions. The secret lies in understanding how protein-rich flours, healthy fats, and fiber work together to create maximum flavor and sustained satisfaction, preventing the crash-and-crave cycle of traditional sweets. You'll discover techniques for achieving rich chocolate depth, perfect cake texture, and bakery-worthy presentation using ingredients that actually nourish your body. Each recipe includes complete nutritional information, glycemic impact ratings, and strategies for mindful portion control that feels abundant rather than restrictive.

List of Recipes

Baked Cinnamon Apple Crisp

8 | 20 minutes | 35 minutes

A warm, comforting dessert featuring tender apples topped with a crunchy almond and oat topping.

DIRECTIONS

1. Preheat oven to 375°F (190°C). Grease 9x9-inch baking dish.
2. In large bowl, toss sliced apples with lemon juice, erythritol, cinnamon, nutmeg, and almond flour.
3. Transfer apple mixture to prepared baking dish.
4. In same bowl, combine oats, almond flour, walnuts, melted coconut oil, maple syrup, cinnamon, and salt.
5. Sprinkle topping evenly over apples.
6. Bake 30-35 minutes until topping is golden brown and apples are tender.
7. Let cool 10 minutes before serving.

NUTRITION

Per serving: 185 calories, 4g protein, 26g carbohydrates, 8g fat, 5g fiber

STORAGE

Keeps for up to 3 days at room temperature or 5 days refrigerated.

INGREDIENTS

For filling:

- 6 medium apples (Honeycrisp or Granny Smith), peeled and sliced
- 2 tablespoons lemon juice
- 2 tablespoons erythritol or coconut sugar
- 1 teaspoon ground cinnamon
- 1/4 teaspoon ground nutmeg
- 1 tablespoon almond flour

For topping:

- 1 cup old-fashioned oats (certified gluten-free)
- 1/2 cup almond flour
- 1/3 cup chopped walnuts
- 3 tablespoons coconut oil, melted
- 2 tablespoons maple syrup
- 1/2 teaspoon cinnamon
- 1/4 teaspoon salt

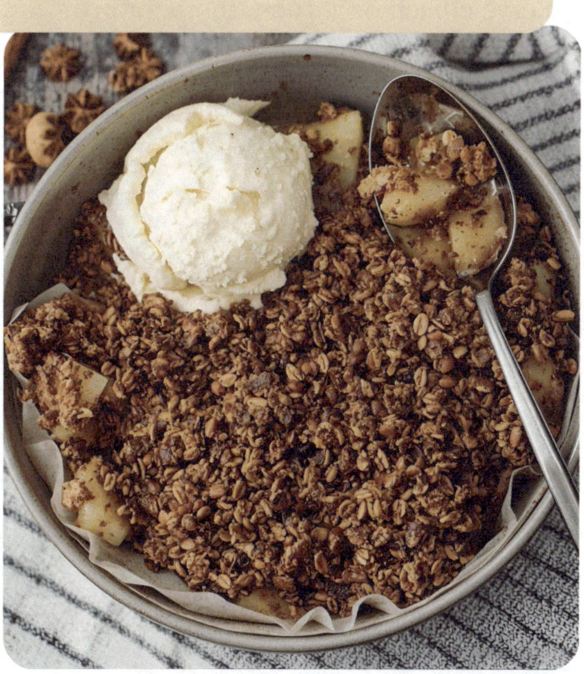

Spiced Poached Pears

INGREDIENTS

- 4 firm Bosc pears, peeled with stems intact
- 2 cups unsweetened apple juice
- 1 cinnamon stick
- 3 whole cloves
- 2 star anise pods
- 1 strip orange zest
- 2 tablespoons honey
- 1 tablespoon lemon juice
- 1/4 cup toasted walnuts, chopped
- 2 tablespoons Greek yogurt (optional)

NUTRITION

Per serving: 145 calories, 2g protein, 32g carbohydrates, 3g fat, 6g fiber

STORAGE

Keeps for up to 3 days refrigerated. Serve chilled or at room temperature.

4 | 15 minutes | 25 minutes

Elegant poached pears infused with warming spices and natural sweetness from fruit juice.

DIRECTIONS

1. Using melon baller or small spoon, remove core from bottom of each pear, leaving stem end intact.
2. In large saucepan, combine apple juice, cinnamon stick, cloves, star anise, orange zest, and honey.
3. Bring to simmer over medium heat.
4. Add pears and cover with parchment paper cut to fit inside pan.
5. Simmer 20-25 minutes, turning pears once, until tender when pierced with knife.
6. Remove pears and set aside.
7. Increase heat to high and reduce poaching liquid by half, about 10 minutes.
8. Strain liquid and stir in lemon juice.
9. Serve pears drizzled with reduced poaching liquid and topped with toasted walnuts.
10. Add dollop of Greek yogurt if desired.

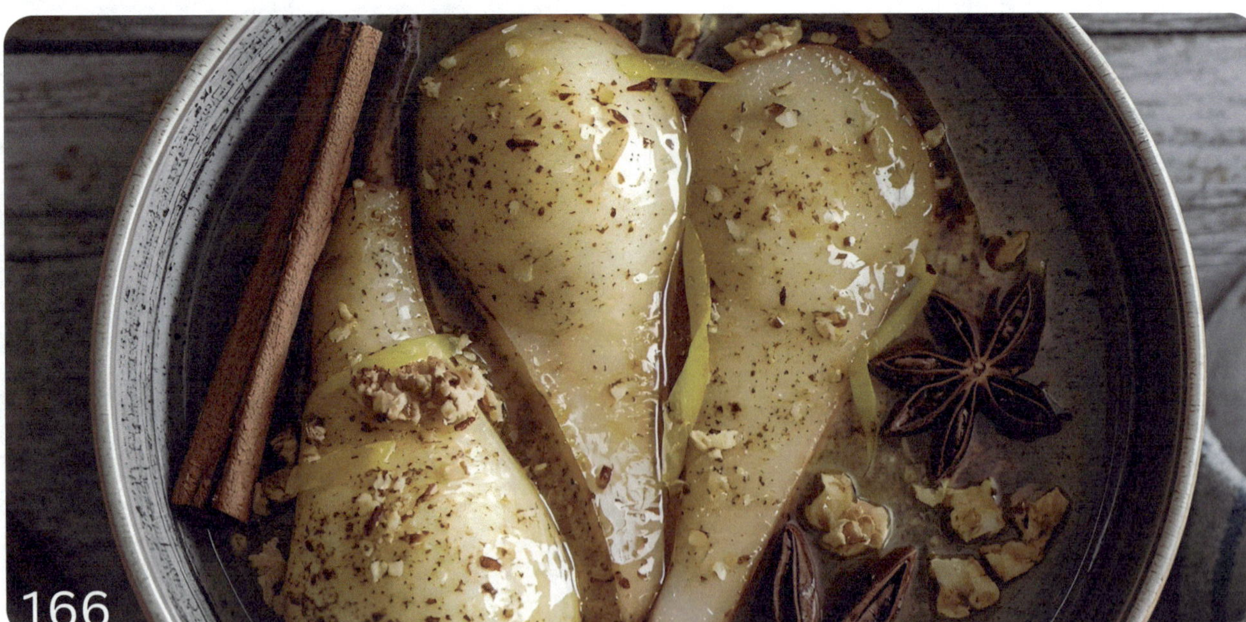

Almond Flour Brownies

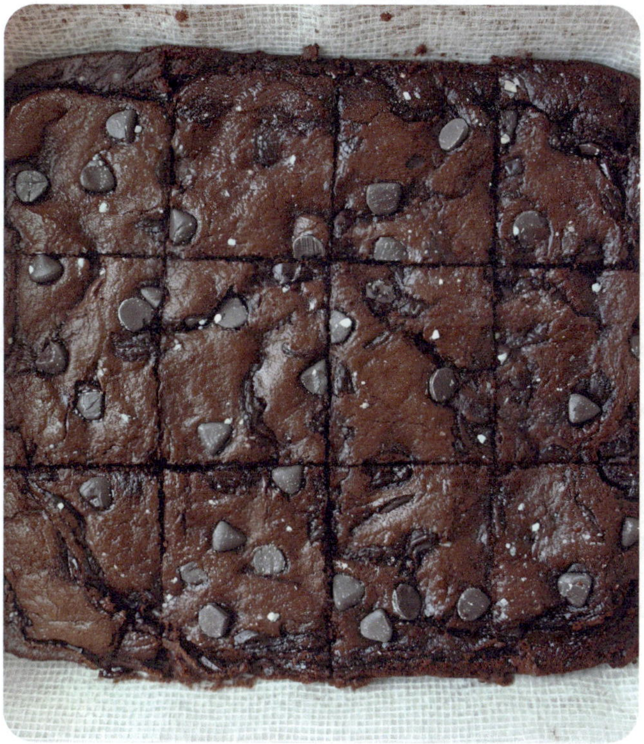

INGREDIENTS

- 2 cups almond flour
- 1/2 cup unsweetened cocoa powder
- 1/2 cup erythritol or coconut sugar
- 1/2 teaspoon baking soda
- 1/2 teaspoon salt
- 1/3 cup coconut oil, melted
- 2 large eggs
- 1/4 cup unsweetened applesauce
- 2 teaspoons vanilla extract
- 1/3 cup dark chocolate chips (85% cacao or higher)
- 1/4 cup chopped walnuts

16 | 15 minutes | 25 minutes

Fudgy, rich brownies made with almond flour that satisfy chocolate cravings without the blood sugar spike.

NUTRITION

Per serving: 105 calories,

4g protein, 9g carbohydrates, 7g fat,

4g fiber

STORAGE

Keep covered at room temperature for 3 days or freeze for up to 3 months

DIRECTION

- Preheat oven to 350°F (175°C). Line 8x8-inch pan with parchment paper.
- In large bowl, whisk together almond flour, cocoa powder, erythritol, baking soda, and salt.
- In another bowl, whisk together melted coconut oil, eggs, applesauce, and vanilla.
- Pour wet ingredients into dry ingredients and stir until just combined.
- Fold in chocolate chips and walnuts.
- Spread batter evenly in prepared pan.
- Bake 20-25 minutes until edges are set and toothpick inserted in center comes out with a few moist crumbs.
- Cool completely in pan before cutting into 16 squares.

Double Chocolate Avocado Pudding

Silky avocado-based pudding with rich chocolate flavor and a healthy twist.

Servings	Prep time	Cook time
6	10 minutes plus 2 hours chilling	0 minutes

INGREDIENTS

- 3 large ripe avocados, peeled and pitted
- ½ cup unsweetened cocoa powder
- ⅓ cup powdered erythritol (or equivalent artificial sweetener)
- ⅓ cup unsweetened almond milk
- 2 tsp pure vanilla extract
- A pinch of salt
- ¼ tsp ground cinnamon (optional)
- 2 tbsp sugar-free mini chocolate chips
- Fresh raspberries or strawberries for garnish
- Chopped toasted walnuts for garnish (optional)

DIRECTIONS

1. In a food processor, combine avocados, cocoa powder, powdered sweetener, almond milk, vanilla, salt, and cinnamon (if using).
2. Process until smooth and creamy, scraping down sides as necessary.
3. Stir in chocolate chips by hand.
4. Divide pudding among 6 serving cups.
5. Cover and chill at least 2 hours to set.
6. Garnish with fresh berries and toasted walnuts (if desired) before serving.

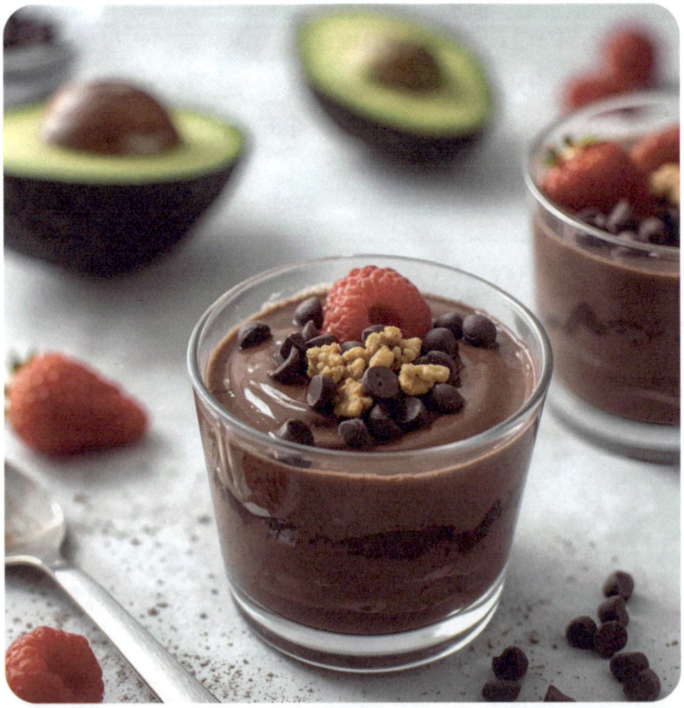

NUTRITION

Per serving: 195 calories, 4g protein, 11g carbohydrates, 8g fat, 8g fiber

STORAGE

Keeps refrigerated for up to 3 days. Cover tightly to prevent browning.

Toasted Almond "Shortbread" Crisps

Crispy almond flour "shortbread" with toasted almonds and a buttery bite.

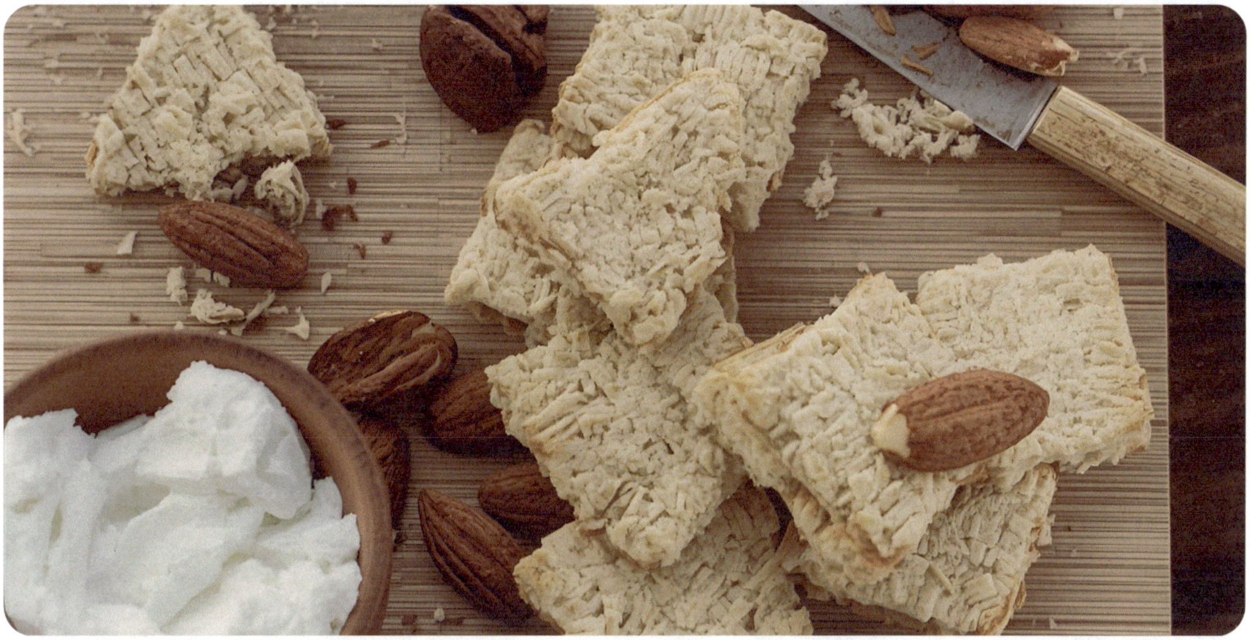

INGREDIENTS

- 1½ cups almond flour
- ¼ cup powdered erythritol (or equivalent artificial sweetener)
- ¼ tsp salt
- ½ tsp vanilla extract
- 3 tbsp melted coconut oil
- 2 tbsp toasted sliced almonds

NUTRITION

Per serving, 3 crisps: 140 calories, 5g protein, 4g carbohydrates, 12g fat, 3g fiber

STORAGE

Keeps in an airtight container for up to 1 week.

Servings	Prep time	Cook time
8	10 minutes	15 minutes

DIRECTIONS

1. Preheat oven to 325°F (160°C). Line a baking sheet with parchment paper.
2. In a bowl, mix almond flour, powdered sweetener, and salt.
3. Stir in vanilla and melted coconut oil until a dough forms.
4. Roll dough between two sheets of parchment to ¼-inch thickness.
5. Remove top parchment. Sprinkle with toasted sliced almonds, gently pressing in.
6. Cut into 2-inch squares (no need to separate).
7. Bake 13–15 minutes until golden around edges.
8. Let cool on the sheet, then break into squares.

Coconut Panna Cotta with Berry Compote

6

20 minutes
(plus 4 hour chilling)

10 minutes

An elegant, creamy dessert with bright berry compote that's naturally dairy-free and refined sugar-free.

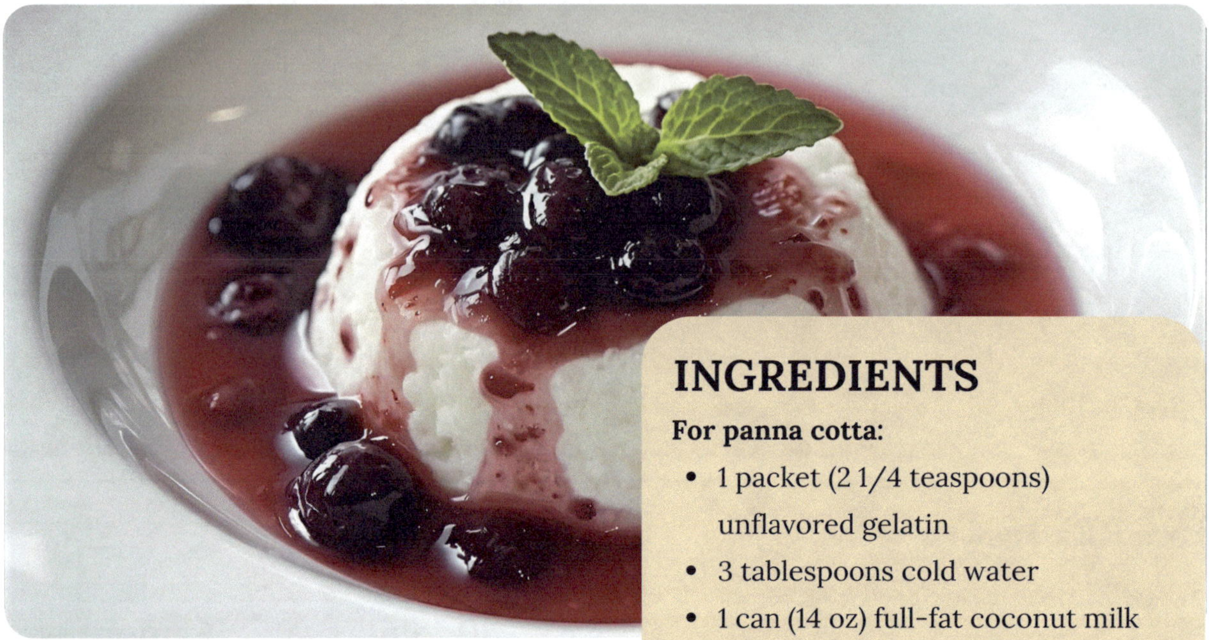

INGREDIENTS

For panna cotta:

- 1 packet (2 1/4 teaspoons) unflavored gelatin
- 3 tablespoons cold water
- 1 can (14 oz) full-fat coconut milk
- 1/3 cup honey
- 1 teaspoon vanilla extract
- 1/4 teaspoon almond extract

For berry compote:

- 2 cups mixed berries (strawberries, blueberries, raspberries)
- 2 tablespoons honey
- 1 tablespoon lemon juice
- 1 teaspoon lemon zest

DIRECTIONS

1. Make panna cotta: Sprinkle gelatin over cold water in small bowl. Let bloom 5 minutes.
2. In saucepan, heat coconut milk and honey over medium heat until just simmering.
3. Remove from heat and whisk in bloomed gelatin until dissolved.
4. Stir in vanilla and almond extracts.
5. Divide among 6 ramekins or glasses. Refrigerate 4 hours until set.
6. Make compote: In small saucepan, combine berries, honey, lemon juice, and zest.
7. Cook over medium heat 8-10 minutes until berries release juices and mixture thickens slightly.
8. Cool completely before serving.
9. Top each panna cotta with berry compote just before serving.

NUTRITION

Per serving: 195 calories, 3g protein, 24g carbohydrates, 11g fat, 3g fiber

STORAGE

Panna cotta keeps for up to 3 days refrigerated. Compote keeps for 5 days.

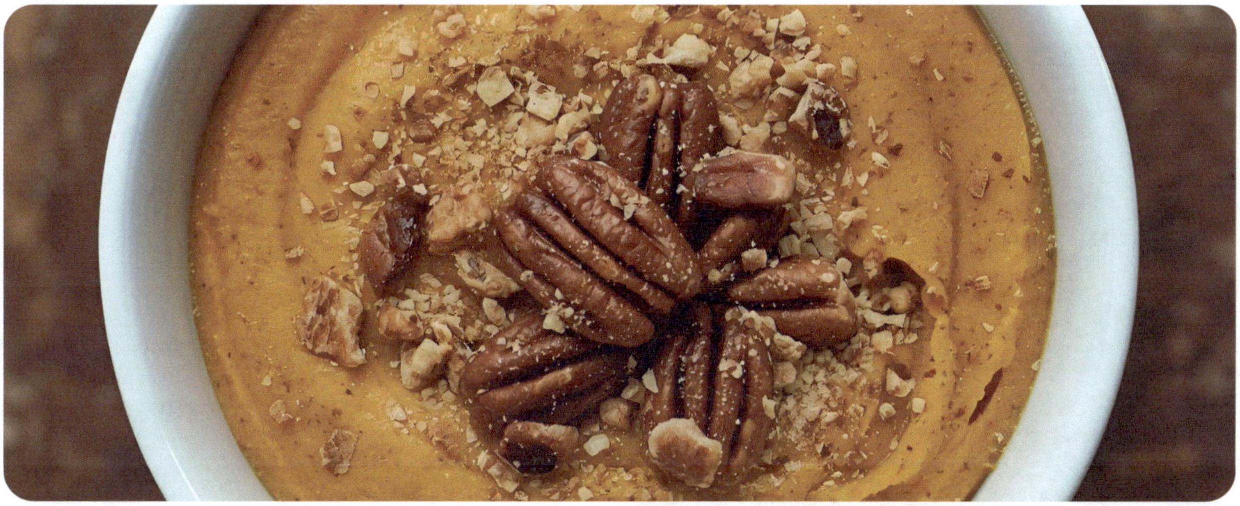

Spiced Pumpkin Mousse

Fluffy pumpkin mousse with warm spices and a dairy-free cream base.

8

10 minutes
(plus 2 hours chilling)

0 minutes

DIRECTIONS

1. In a bowl, mix pumpkin puree, powdered sweetener, cinnamon, ginger, nutmeg, and salt until well combined.
2. In another bowl, whip the coconut cream and vanilla until thick and fluffy.
3. Gently fold the pumpkin mixture into the whipped coconut cream.
4. Divide among 8 glasses or bowls.
5. Chill at least 2 hours.
6. Garnish with candied pecans or crushed graham cracker (optional).

INGREDIENTS

- 2 cups pumpkin puree (fresh or canned)
- ½ cup powdered erythritol (or equivalent artificial sweetener)
- 1 tsp ground cinnamon
- ½ tsp ground ginger
- ¼ tsp ground nutmeg
- A pinch of salt
- 2 cups refrigerated coconut cream (the thick part from full-fat canned coconut milk, chilled overnight)
- 1 tsp vanilla extract
- Candied pecans or crushed graham crackers (optional, for garnish)

NUTRITION

Per serving: 130 calories, 1g protein, 7g carbohydrates, 11g fat, 2g fiber

STORAGE

Keeps refrigerated for up to 3 days.

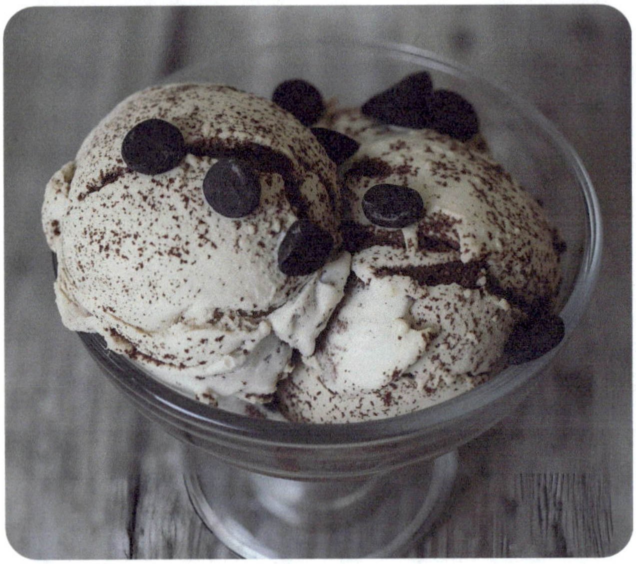

Mocha Frozen "Yogurt"

Dairy-free frozen yogurt infused with cocoa and espresso for a mocha kick.

Servings	Prep time	Cook time
6	10 minutes (plus 4 hours freezing)	0 minutes

INGREDIENTS

- 3 cups unsweetened coconut yogurt
- ½ cup powdered erythritol (or equivalent artificial sweetener)
- 2 tbsp unsweetened cocoa powder
- 1 tsp instant espresso powder
- 1 tsp vanilla extract
- 2 tbsp dark chocolate chips (optional, for garnish)

DIRECTIONS

1. In a food processor, blend coconut yogurt, powdered sweetener, cocoa powder, espresso powder, and vanilla until smooth.
2. Pour mixture into a freezer-safe container.
3. Cover and freeze 4 hours, stirring every 30 minutes for a creamy texture.
4. Scoop into bowls and top with chocolate chips before serving.

NUTRITION

Per serving: 125 calories, 2g protein, 8g carbohydrates, 9g fat, 2g fiber

STORAGE

Keeps frozen for up to 2 weeks.

Banana "Ice Cream" Sundaes

4	5 minutes	0 minutes

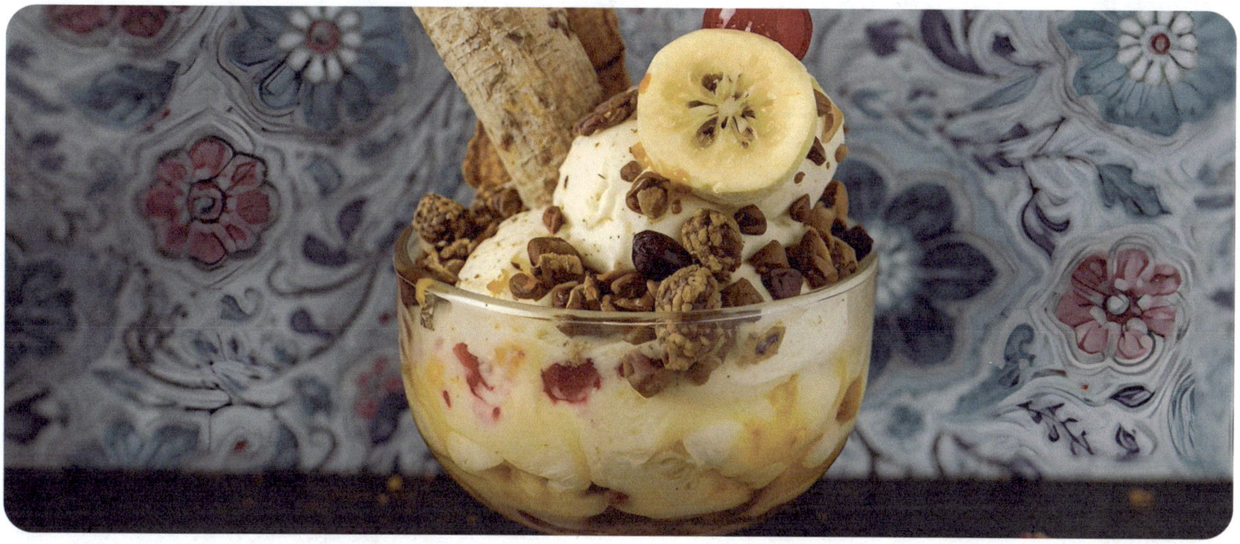

Frozen bananas blended into creamy "ice cream" topped with chocolate and nuts.

DIRECTIONS

1. In a food processor, blend frozen bananas, peanut butter, cinnamon, and vanilla until smooth and creamy, scraping down sides as needed.
2. Scoop into bowls.
3. Top with chocolate chips, toasted walnuts, and a dollop of whipped coconut cream (if using).
4. Serve immediately.

NUTRITION

Per serving: 150 calories, 3g protein, 22g carbohydrates, 6g fat, 3g fiber

STORAGE

Best served fresh, but can be refrozen for up to 3 days (let soften before eating).

INGREDIENTS

- 4 ripe bananas, peeled, sliced, and frozen
- 2 tbsp peanut butter or almond butter
- ½ tsp ground cinnamon
- ⅛ tsp pure vanilla extract
- 2 tbsp sugar-free chocolate chips or chopped dark chocolate (85% cacao)
- 2 tbsp toasted chopped walnuts (optional)
- 2 tbsp whipped coconut cream (optional, see recipe notes)

Cheesecake-Stuffed Strawberries

8 (16 strawberries) | 15 minutes | 0 minutes

Juicy strawberries filled with sweet, creamy cheesecake and a touch of coconut.

INGREDIENTS

- 16 large strawberries, hulled and cored (keep intact)
- 8 oz cream cheese, softened (or dairy-free cream cheese alternative)
- ¼ cup powdered erythritol (or equivalent artificial sweetener)
- 1 tsp pure vanilla extract
- 1 tbsp unsweetened shredded coconut (optional, for garnish)

DIRECTIONS

1. In a bowl, beat cream cheese or alternative with sweetener and vanilla until smooth and creamy.
2. Spoon or pipe filling into each strawberry.
3. Sprinkle with shredded coconut (if using).
4. Serve immediately or chill until ready to serve.

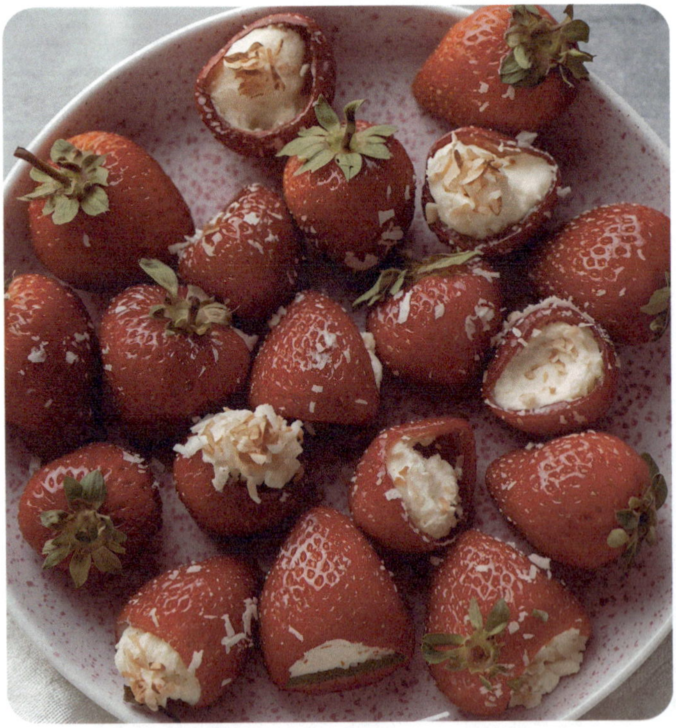

NUTRITION

Per serving: 105 calories, 4g protein, 9g carbohydrates, 7g fat, 4g fiber

STORAGE

Keep covered at room temperature for 3 days or freeze for up to 3 months

Dark Chocolate Almond Bark

16

15 minutes (plus 1 hour setting)

0 minutes

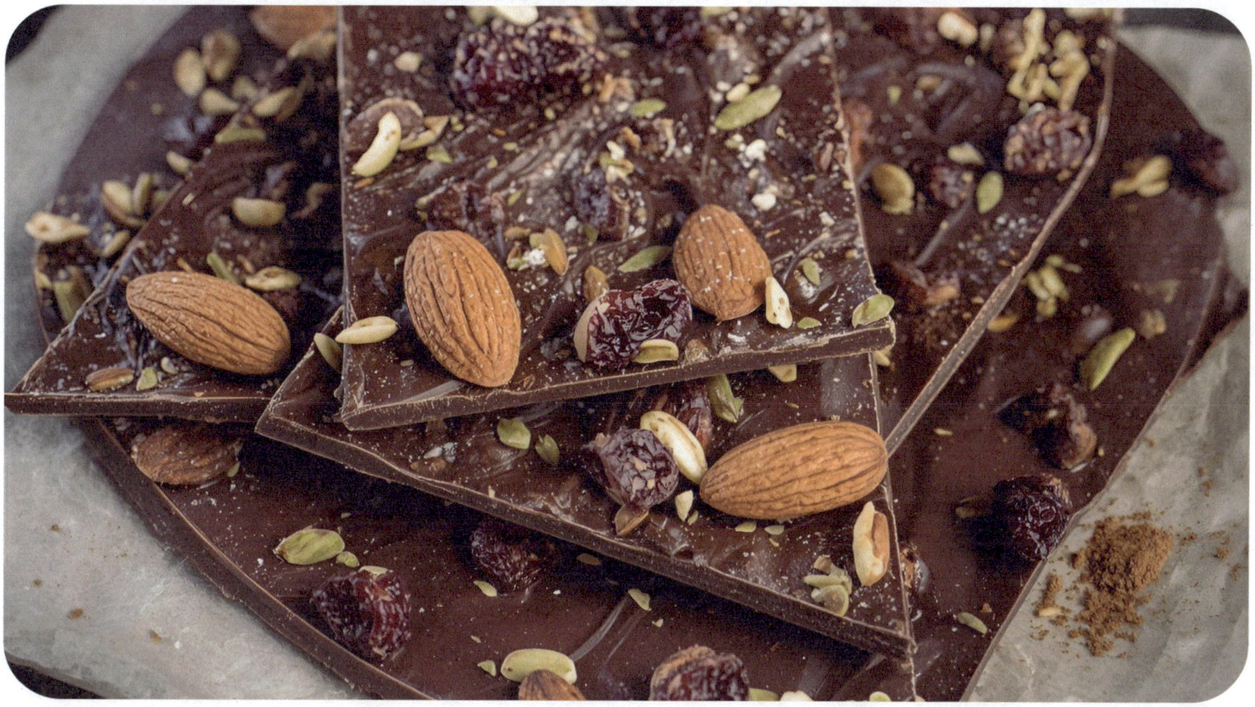

Sophisticated chocolate bark studded with nuts and seeds for the perfect portion-controlled treat.

INGREDIENTS

- 8 oz dark chocolate (85% cacao or higher), chopped
- 1/2 cup raw almonds, roughly chopped
- 1/4 cup pumpkin seeds
- 2 tablespoons dried cranberries (no sugar added)
- 1 tablespoon chia seeds
- 1/2 teaspoon sea salt flakes
- 1/4 teaspoon cinnamon

DIRECTIONS

1. Line 8x8-inch pan with parchment paper.
2. Melt chocolate in double boiler or microwave in 30-second intervals, stirring until smooth.
3. Pour melted chocolate into prepared pan and spread evenly.
4. Immediately sprinkle with almonds, pumpkin seeds, cranberries, chia seeds, sea salt, and cinnamon.
5. Gently press toppings into chocolate.
6. Refrigerate 1 hour until completely set.
7. Break into 16 irregular pieces.

NUTRITION

Per piece: 95 calories, 3g protein, 6g carbohydrates, 7g fat, 2g fiber

STORAGE

Store in airtight container in refrigerator for up to 2 weeks or freeze for 3 months.

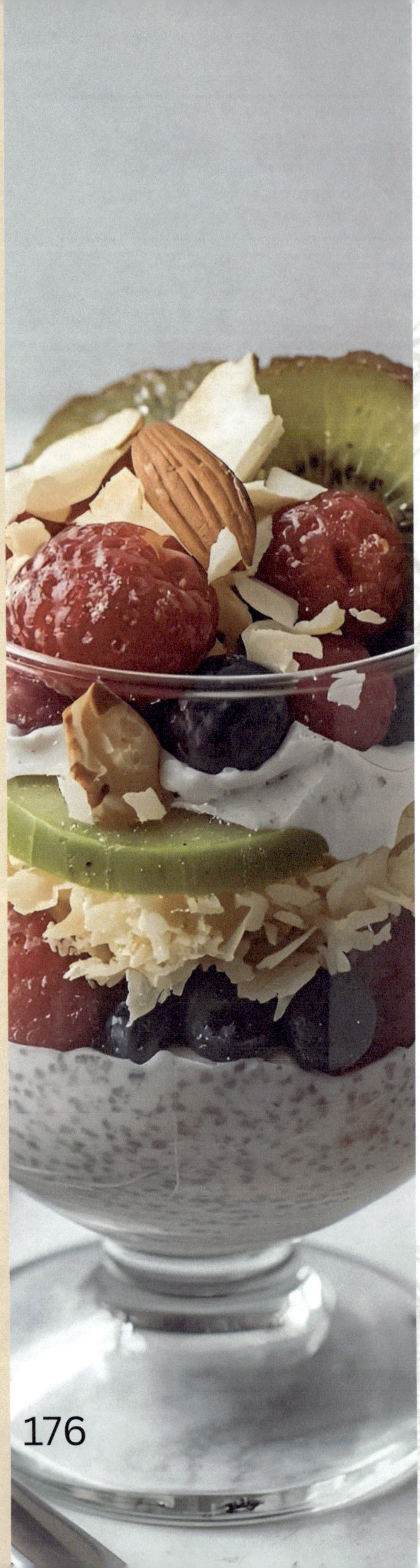

TIPS FOR GUILT-FREE DESSERT SUCCESS

Natural Sweetness First: Let fruit provide primary sweetness whenever possible. Ripe bananas, dates, applesauce, and berries add sweetness plus fiber, vitamins, and antioxidants.

Embrace Healthy Fats: Nuts, seeds, avocados, and coconut provide richness and satisfaction that make smaller portions feel indulgent.

Protein Power: Include protein through nuts, seeds, Greek yogurt, or protein powder to slow sugar absorption and increase satiety.

Spice for Interest: Cinnamon, vanilla, cardamom, and other warm spices enhance perceived sweetness without adding calories or affecting blood sugar.

Portion Mindfully: These desserts are designed to satisfy in smaller portions. Use small bowls, ramekins, or glasses to create appropriate serving sizes.

Texture Matters: Combine smooth and crunchy elements for more interesting eating experiences that feel more satisfying.

Make-Ahead Advantages: Many of these desserts actually improve with time as flavors develop and textures set properly.

Quality Chocolate: When using chocolate, choose varieties with 70% cacao or higher for less sugar and more antioxidants.

Fresh Finish: Add fresh fruit, herbs, or nuts just before serving to maintain optimal textures and brightest flavors.

Storage Wisdom: Most of these desserts keep well refrigerated, making them perfect for meal prep or entertaining preparation.

Remember that the goal of guilt-free desserts isn't to perfectly replicate traditional sweets, but to create new favorites that satisfy your desire for something sweet while supporting your health goals. When desserts are this naturally delicious and nutritious, smaller portions provide more satisfaction than larger servings of less wholesome alternatives

CHAPTER 15

Emergency Meals & Pantry Rescues

Life doesn't always cooperate with our meal planning, no matter how organized we try to be. The refrigerator runs empty the night before grocery shopping, unexpected guests arrive, or a busy week leaves you staring at a collection of random ingredients wondering how to turn them into dinner. These moments can feel particularly challenging when managing both celiac disease and diabetes, where you can't simply order pizza or grab whatever's convenient at the corner store.

List of Recipes

1. Missing Eggs: Chickpea Flour Power Pancakes
2. No Fresh Vegetables: Mediterranean White Bean Stew
3. Out of Fresh Protein: Smoky Lentil Walnut "Meatballs"
4. Almond Flour Rescue: Crispy Herb Crackers
5. Coconut Flour Last Call: Chocolate Mug Cake

This chapter is your safety net for when fresh ingredients run low but your commitment to nourishing meals remains strong. These aren't desperate measures—they're genuine solutions that often become favorite discoveries.

Building Your Emergency Pantry

Protein Foundations: Canned wild salmon, sardines, and tuna provide omega-3 rich proteins. Eggs keep for weeks and transform into everything from scrambles to baked goods. Nuts, seeds, and nut butters offer protein and healthy fats. Canned beans (rinsed to reduce sodium) provide plant-based protein and fiber.

Vegetable Insurance: Frozen vegetables often retain more nutrients than stored fresh vegetables and never go bad unexpectedly. Keep broccoli, spinach, mixed bell peppers, and cauliflower rice. Canned tomatoes and jarred roasted red peppers add depth to many dishes.

Flexible Starches: Brown rice, quinoa, and gluten-free oats provide satisfying meal bases. Sweet potatoes keep for weeks in a cool, dark place. Frozen cauliflower rice offers a lower-carb alternative.

The Art of Creative Substitution

Missing Fresh Herbs? Use one-third the amount of dried herbs, adding them earlier in cooking.

Out of Fresh Vegetables? Frozen vegetables substitute for fresh—add them toward the end to prevent mushiness. Canned vegetables work well in soups and stews.

No Fresh Protein? Canned fish, eggs, nuts, and legumes replace fresh meat. Canned salmon becomes salmon cakes or protein-rich salad toppings.

Limited Fresh Dairy? Canned coconut milk or nutritional yeast provide richness. Blend nuts and seeds with water to create cream-like sauce bases.

Extending Ingredient Life

Toast almond flour lightly to refresh flavor. Roast softening vegetables to concentrate flavors. Process wilting herbs into pestos. Cook overripe fruits into sugar-free compotes.

Missing Eggs: Chickpea Flour Power Pancakes

When you're out of eggs but craving breakfast, chickpea flour creates surprisingly fluffy, protein-rich pancakes that satisfy morning hunger while keeping blood sugar stable.

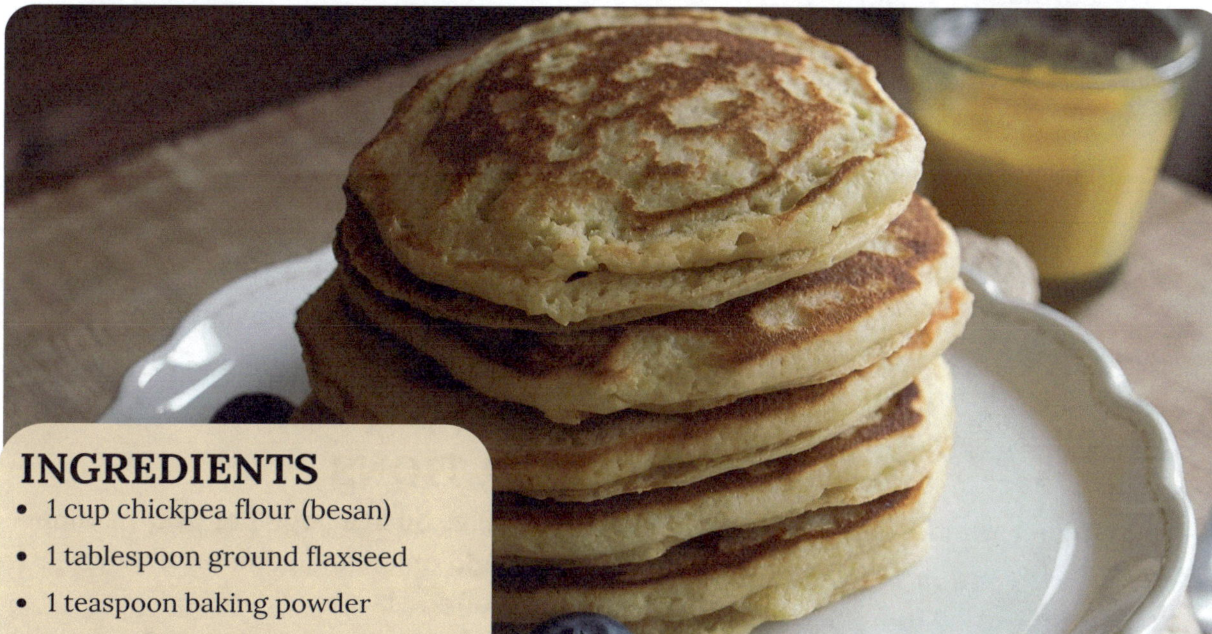

INGREDIENTS

- 1 cup chickpea flour (besan)
- 1 tablespoon ground flaxseed
- 1 teaspoon baking powder
- 1/2 teaspoon salt
- 1/4 teaspoon turmeric (for color)
- 1 1/4 cups unsweetened almond milk
- 2 tablespoons olive oil
- 1 teaspoon vanilla extract
- 1/2 teaspoon liquid stevia (or to taste)
- Cooking spray
- Optional: 1/4 cup blueberries or chopped nuts

4	5 minutes	10 minutes

DIRECTIONS

1. In a medium bowl, whisk together chickpea flour, flaxseed, baking powder, salt, and turmeric.
2. In a separate bowl, combine almond milk, olive oil, vanilla extract, and stevia.
3. Pour wet ingredients into dry ingredients and whisk until just combined. Let batter rest for 2-3 minutes to thicken.
4. Heat a non-stick pan or griddle over medium heat. Spray with cooking spray.
5. Pour 1/4 cup batter per pancake onto hot griddle. Add berries or nuts if using.
6. Cook for 2-3 minutes until edges are set and bubbles form on surface. Flip and cook 1-2 minutes more until golden.
7. Serve immediately with sugar-free syrup or fresh fruit.

NUTRITION

Per Serving: 145 calories, 6g protein, 14g carbohydrates, 8g fat, 4g fiber

STORAGE

Leftover pancakes freeze well for up to 3 months. Reheat in toaster or oven.

No Fresh Vegetables: Mediterranean White Bean Rescue Stew

6 | 10 minutes | 25 minutes

This hearty stew transforms pantry staples into a deeply satisfying meal that proves canned and frozen ingredients can create restaurant-quality results.

INGREDIENTS

- 2 tablespoons olive oil
- 1 large onion, diced (or 2 tablespoons dried minced onion)
- 4 cloves garlic, minced (or 1 teaspoon garlic powder)
- 1 teaspoon dried oregano
- 1/2 teaspoon dried thyme
- 1/4 teaspoon red pepper flakes
- 1 can (14.5 oz) diced tomatoes, undrained
- 2 tablespoons tomato paste
- 3 cups vegetable broth (low-sodium)
- 2 cans (15 oz each) cannellini beans, drained and rinsed
- 2 cups frozen spinach, thawed and drained
- 1 cup frozen artichoke hearts (optional)
- 1/4 cup sun-dried tomatoes, chopped (oil-packed, drained)
- 2 tablespoons lemon juice
- Salt and black pepper to taste
- 1/4 cup fresh parsley, chopped (or 1 tablespoon dried)

DIRECTIONS

1. Heat olive oil in a large pot over medium heat. Add onion and cook for 5 minutes until softened.
2. Add garlic, oregano, thyme, and red pepper flakes. Cook for 1 minute until fragrant.
3. Stir in diced tomatoes, tomato paste, and vegetable broth. Bring to a simmer.
4. Add cannellini beans and sun-dried tomatoes. Simmer for 15 minutes to blend flavors.
5. Stir in spinach and artichoke hearts. Cook for 3-5 minutes until heated through.
6. Remove from heat and stir in lemon juice. Season with salt and pepper to taste.
7. Garnish with parsley before serving. Serve with gluten-free crackers or over quinoa if desired.

NUTRITION

Per serving: 185 calories, 9g protein, 28g carbohydrates, 5g fat, 9g fiber

STORAGE

Refrigerate for up to 5 days or freeze for up to 3 months. Add a splash of broth when reheating if needed.

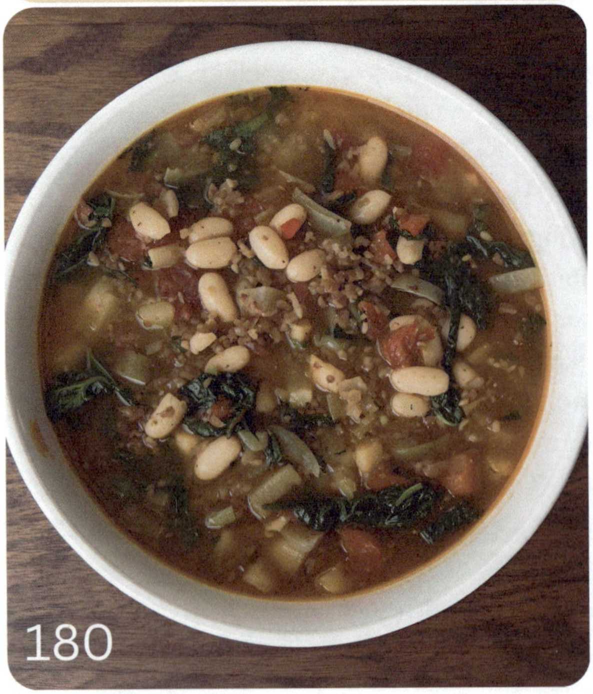

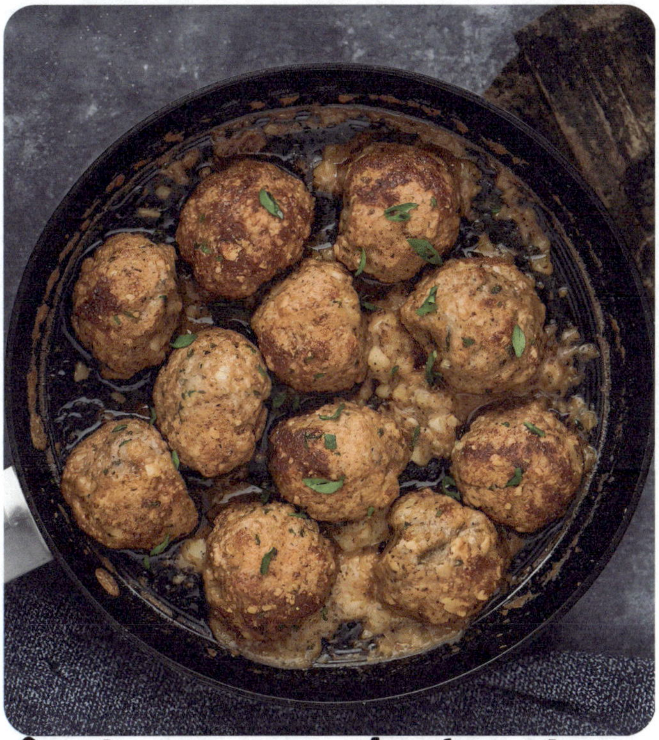

Out of Fresh Protein: Smoky Lentil Walnut "Meatballs"

These protein-rich "meatballs" use pantry staples to create a satisfying main dish that works over pasta, in soup, or as appetizers.

4	15 minutes	20 minutes

NUTRITION

Per serving, 4 meatballs: 235 calories, 11g protein, 18g carbohydrates, 14g fat, 8g fiber

STORAGE

Refrigerate for up to 5 days or freeze for up to 3 months. Reheat in oven or microwave.

INGREDIENTS

- 1 cup cooked brown lentils (from 1/2 cup dried, or 1 can drained)
- 3/4 cup walnuts, finely chopped
- 1/2 cup gluten-free breadcrumbs (or ground oats)
- 1/4 cup ground flaxseed
- 1/4 cup nutritional yeast
- 2 tablespoons tomato paste
- 1 tablespoon olive oil
- 1 teaspoon smoked paprika
- 1/2 teaspoon garlic powder
- 1/2 teaspoon onion powder
- 1/2 teaspoon dried oregano
- 1/2 teaspoon salt
- 1/4 teaspoon black pepper
- 2-3 tablespoons vegetable broth (as needed)
- Cooking spray

DIRECTION

1. Preheat oven to 375°F (190°C). Line a baking sheet with parchment paper.
2. If using dried lentils, cook according to package directions until tender. Drain and cool slightly.
3. In a large bowl, mash half the lentils with a fork, leaving some texture.
4. Add remaining whole lentils, walnuts, breadcrumbs, flaxseed, nutritional yeast, tomato paste, olive oil, and all seasonings.
5. Mix well. If mixture is too dry, add vegetable broth 1 tablespoon at a time until mixture holds together when squeezed.
6. Form mixture into 16 walnut-sized balls and place on prepared baking sheet.
7. Spray lightly with cooking spray and bake for 18-20 minutes, turning once halfway through, until golden and firm.
8. Serve immediately or store for later use.

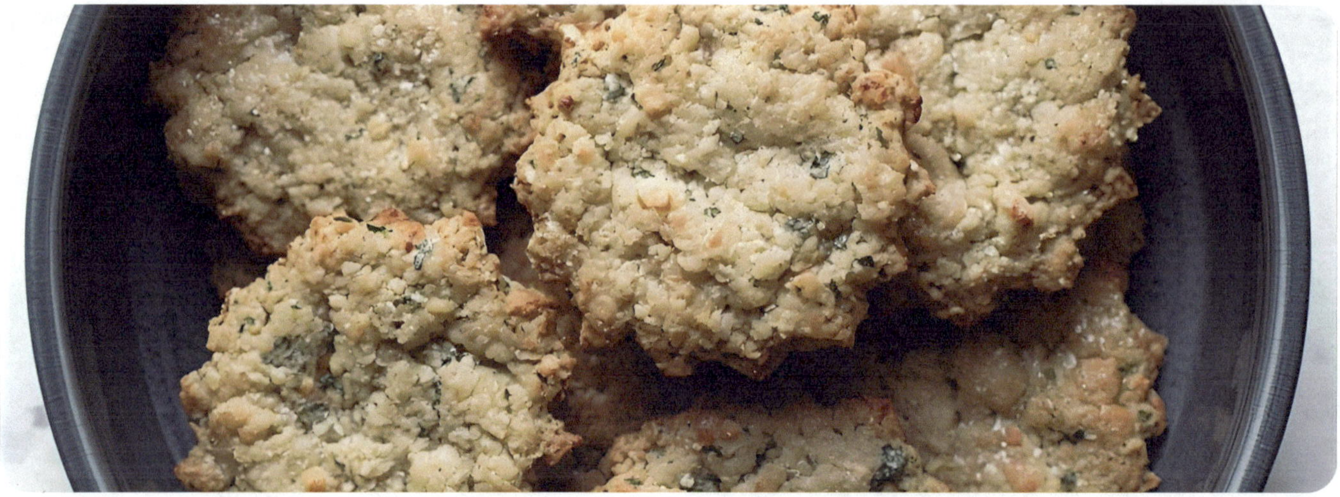

Using Up Soon-to-Expire Ingredients

Almond Flour Rescue: Crispy Herb Crackers

Servings	Prep time	Cook time
8 (about 32 crackers)	10 minutes	15 minutes

INGREDIENTS

- 2 cups almond flour
- 1/2 teaspoon salt
- 1/2 teaspoon garlic powder
- 1/2 teaspoon dried herbs (rosemary, thyme, or Italian seasoning)
- 1/4 teaspoon black pepper
- 2 tablespoons olive oil
- 1 large egg
- 1-2 tablespoons water (if needed)
- Coarse sea salt for sprinkling

Transform almond flour that's approaching its expiration date into crispy, satisfying crackers that store well and provide emergency snack options.

DIRECTIONS

1. Preheat oven to 350°F (175°C). Line a large baking sheet with parchment paper.
2. In a bowl, combine almond flour, salt, garlic powder, herbs, and pepper.
3. Add olive oil and egg, mixing until dough forms. Add water if mixture is too dry.
4. Place dough between two sheets of parchment paper and roll to 1/8-inch thickness.
5. Remove top parchment and transfer bottom sheet with dough to baking sheet.
6. Score into 2-inch squares with a knife. Sprinkle with coarse salt.
7. Bake for 12-15 minutes until golden brown and crispy.
8. Cool completely before breaking apart along scored lines.

NUTRITION

Per serving, 4 crackers: 165 calories, 6g protein, 5g carbohydrates, 14g fat, 3g fiber

STORAGE

Store in airtight container for up to 1 week.

Coconut Flour Last Call: Chocolate Mug Cake

Servings	Prep time	Cook time
1	3 minutes	90 seconds

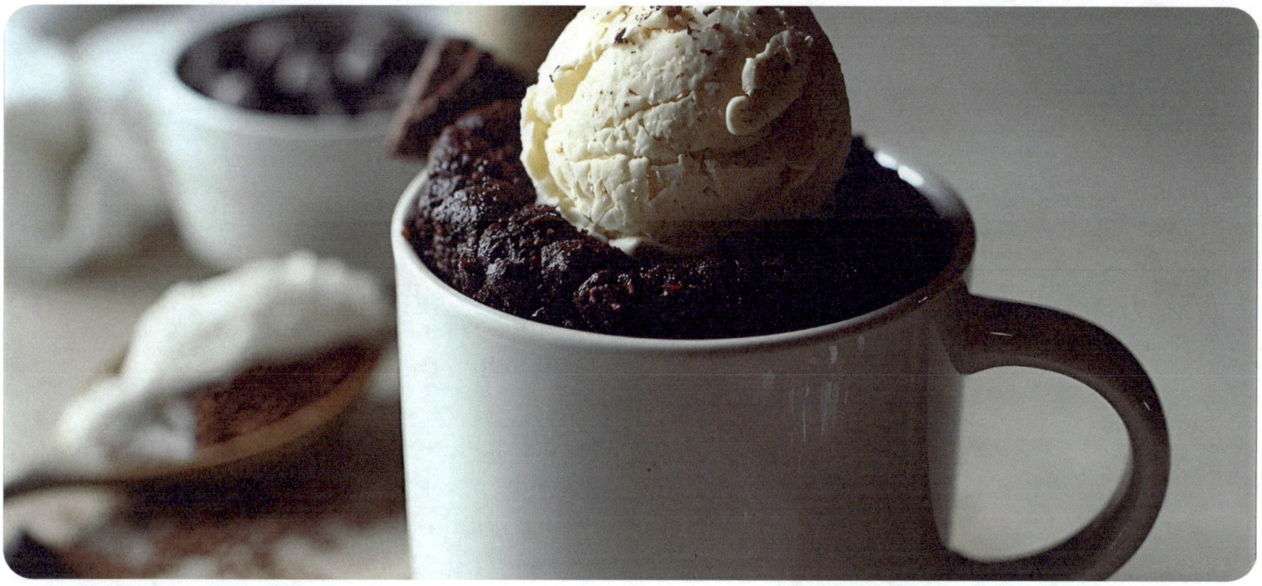

Use up the last of your coconut flour in this satisfying single-serving dessert that's ready in under 5 minutes.

INGREDIENTS

- 2 tablespoons coconut flour
- 1 tablespoon unsweetened cocoa powder
- 1/4 teaspoon baking powder
- Pinch of salt
- 1/4 teaspoon vanilla extract
- 1/4 teaspoon liquid stevia (or to taste)
- 1 large egg
- 2 tablespoons unsweetened almond milk
- 1 tablespoon coconut oil, melted
- 1 tablespoon sugar-free chocolate chips (optional)

DIRECTIONS

1. In a microwave-safe mug, whisk together coconut flour, cocoa powder, baking powder, and salt.
2. In a small bowl, whisk together vanilla, stevia, egg, almond milk, and melted coconut oil.
3. Pour wet ingredients into mug and stir until completely combined. Fold in chocolate chips if using.
4. Microwave for 60-90 seconds until cake springs back when lightly touched.
5. Let cool for 1 minute before eating. Serve with fresh berries if desired.

NUTRITION

Per serving: 195 calories, 8g protein, 9g carbohydrates, 15g fat, 6g fiber

STORAGE

Best consumed immediately, but can be refrigerated overnight and reheated briefly.

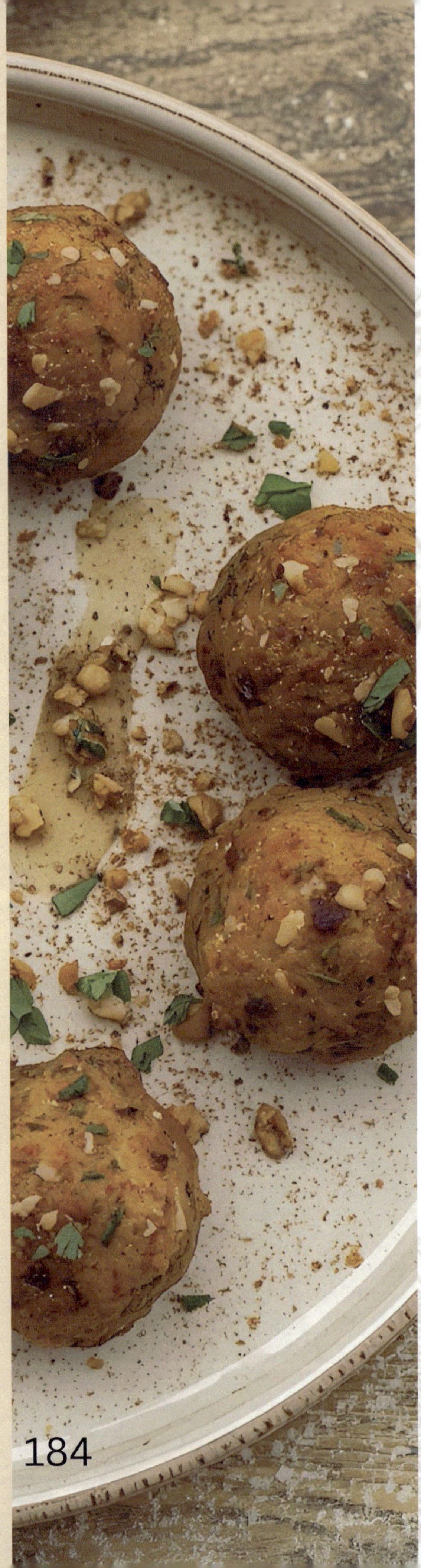

EMERGENCY MEAL PLANNING STRATEGY

The 5-Ingredient Challenge: Keep a running list of 5-ingredient meals you can make entirely from pantry staples. Examples include: quinoa + canned beans + frozen vegetables + olive oil + lemon juice, or eggs + frozen spinach + cheese + tomatoes + herbs.

Rotation System: Use ingredients in order of their expiration dates, not in order of preference. Mark purchase dates on gluten-free flours and alternative sweeteners to ensure you use them while they're fresh.

Flavor Boosters: Keep small amounts of high-impact ingredients that can transform simple combinations: good olive oil, citrus, vinegar, hot sauce, herbs, and spices. These turn basic protein-and-vegetable combinations into satisfying meals.

One-Pot Solutions: Master a few one-pot meals that can be adapted based on available ingredients. A basic formula of protein + vegetables + liquid + seasonings can become soup, stew, curry, or grain bowl depending on proportions and spices used.

Backup Planning: Always keep ingredients for 2-3 complete meals that require no fresh ingredients. Write these recipes on cards and keep them visible in your kitchen so you don't have to think creatively when you're tired or stressed.

Remember that emergency cooking isn't about settling for less -- it's about discovering how resourcefulness and creativity can lead to surprisingly satisfying meals. Some of your favorite recipes might come from these moments when you had to work with what you had rather than what you planned.

Dedication

When I decided to write The Celiabetic Kitchen, I instinctively turned to my bookshelves for inspiration, scanning the stacks of cookbooks that have accumulated over the years. But as I pulled book after book from the shelves, I discovered something unexpected: these weren't just cookbooks—they were the chapters of my life, lovingly gifted by my dearest friend Kathy over thirty years of birthday celebrations.

We met in sixth grade, never imagining that our friendship would endure for more than four decades. As I arranged these cookbooks chronologically, our shared history unfolded like a beautiful memoir: The I Hate to Cook Book during my first apartment days, The Newlywed Cookbook when I married, and volumes on baby food when children arrived—each choice so thoughtful, so perfectly timed to meet me exactly where I was.

But it was during life's challenging chapters that Kathy's gift-giving revealed the true depth of her friendship. When I was diagnosed with celiac disease, that birthday brought carefully researched gluten-free cookbooks. Years later, when diabetes entered the picture, she responded with books on blood sugar management and low-glycemic cooking. These gifts said, "I see you, I believe in you, and I know you'll figure this out."

Now, as I look back, I realize this cookbook represents the culmination of all those birthday gifts. Every technique I've mastered, every successful substitution I've discovered, every moment of joy I've found in my adapted kitchen—all of it built upon the foundation Kathy provided, one year at a time.

The Celiabetic Kitchen exists because of thirty years of thoughtful gifts, but more importantly, it exists because of a friendship that modeled the very principles this cookbook promotes: adaptability, creativity, and the understanding that apparent limitations often become gateways to discoveries we never would have made otherwise.
To Kathy: thank you for teaching me that the most meaningful gifts say, "I see where you are right now, and I believe in where you're going." Thank you for helping me understand that life's unexpected challenges often become its greatest blessings when we have friends who walk beside us.

This cookbook—and the confidence, creativity, and joy it represents—would not exist without you.

With all my love and gratitude,

Gloria

Recipe List

Made in the USA
Monee, IL
14 September 2026

62980072R00103